InStyle
Ultimate
Beauty Secrets

INSTYLE

EDITORIAL
Managing Editor Ariel Foxman
Creative Director Rina Stone
Deputy Managing Editor Lisa Arbetter
Assistant Managing Editor Patrick Moffitt
Director of Photography Marie Suter
Deputy Editors Nancy Bilyeau, Donna Bulseco
Editorial Operations Director Lavinel Savu

Beauty Director Amy Synnott-D'Annibale
Senior Beauty Editor Patricia Alfonso Tortolani
Beauty Editor Kahlana Barfield

Copy Chief Marcia Lawther
Deputy Copy Chief Sandra Vernet

Chief of Reporters DeLora E. Jones
Deputy Chief of Reporters Subira Shaw

Associate Production Manager Bijal Saraiya

Imaging Manager Steven Cadicamo

Executive Director, Public Relations
Beth A. Mitchell

InStyle.com Editor Rosie Amodio

PUBLISHING
Publisher Connie Anne Phillips
Vice President, Finance Maria Tucci Beckett
Associate Publisher, Marketing Ron Prince
Associate Publisher, Advertising
Timothy R. O'Connor
Vice President, Consumer Marketing
Holley Cavanna
Executive Director, Consumer Marketing
Stephanie Chan

ULTIMATE BEAUTY SECRETS
Editor Isabel González Whitaker
Special Projects Editor Brett Hill
Copy Editor Margaret Rauch
Reporter Rachel Williams
Photo Editor Rebecca Karamehmedovic
Editorial Assistant Elisabeth Durkin

TIME HOME ENTERTAINMENT
Publisher Richard Fraiman
General Manager Steven Sandonato
Executive Director, Marketing Services
Carol Pittard
Director, Retail & Special Sales Tom Mifsud
Director, New Product Development
Peter Harper
Director, Bookazine Development & Marketing
Laura Adam
Publishing Director, Brand Marketing
Joy Butts
Assistant General Counsel Helen Wan
Design & Prepress Manager
Anne-Michelle Gallero
Book Production Manager Susan Chodakiewicz
Associate Manager, Product Marketing
Nina Fleishman

Time Home Entertainment would also like to
thank: Christine Austin, Jeremy Biloon, Glenn
Buonocore, Jim Childs, Rose Cirrincione,
Jacqueline Fitzgerald, Carrie Frazier, Lauren Hall,
Suzanne Janso, Malena Jones, Brynn Joyce, Mona
Li, Robert Marasco, Amy Migliaccio, Kimberly
Posa, Brooke Reger, Dave Rozzelle, Ilene Schreider,
Adriana Tierno, Alex Voznesenskiy, Sydney Webber

MELCHER MEDIA
This book was produced by Melcher Media, Inc.
124 West 13th St.
New York, NY 10011
www.melcher.com

Publisher Charles Melcher
Associate Publisher Bonnie Eldon
Editor in Chief Duncan Bock

Executive Editor Lia Ronnen
Project Editor Lauren Nathan
Production Director Kurt Andrews
Production Assistant Daniel del Valle
Editorial Assistant Coco Joly

InStyle
Ultimate Beauty Secrets

The Best Tips, Tricks, and Shortcuts to Create Your Perfect Look

By the editors of *InStyle*, with Eleni Gage

Designed by Maryjane Fahey Design

InStyle

 Time
HOME ENTERTAINMENT

 MELCHER MEDIA

PRODUCED BY MELCHER MEDIA FOR *INSTYLE*® AND TIME HOME ENTERTAINMENT INC.

Foreword

Every day, *InStyle* editors are showered with precious gems and nuggets of gold. No, our offices don't gleam like the Emerald City, and our staff isn't the most over-accessorized, blingy bunch in the business. What we've got is a treasure trove of wisdom, which we've amassed while doing research for our beauty stories. Our ace team, headed by Beauty Director Amy Synnott-D'Annibale, spends its workdays interviewing dermatologists, makeup artists, perfumers, dentists, manicurists, and others, tapping into their knowledge and know-how and then translating it into information that's useful for you. This may not be the kind of wealth you stash in a safety deposit box, but it is valuable, which is why we wanted to collect it all in one place.

This book is like having all those experts on speed dial. Read it cover to cover and you'll discover things you didn't even know you wanted to know, like the secret to making legs look slimmer with shimmer, and new uses for your cracked eye shadow crumbs. Or refer to it when you're looking for something specific, such as how to prevent wrinkles, which cheek color is right for you, or what you can do to keep lipstick from bleeding.

The tips are timeless and cover every skin type, tone, issue, and beauty personality, so be sure to pass them on to friends and family. After all, nothing feels quite as beautiful as sharing the wealth.

ARIEL FOXMAN
Managing Editor, *InStyle*

Contents

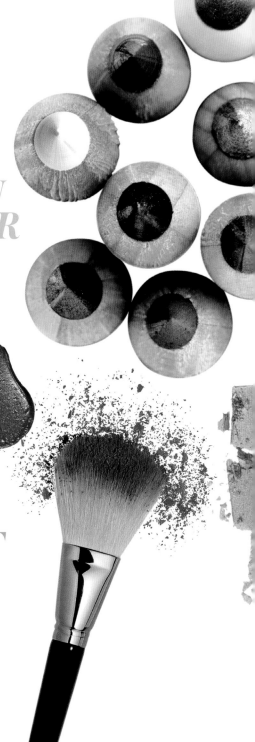

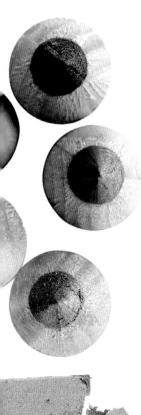

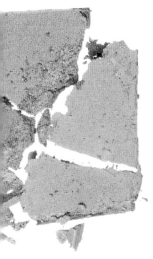

Whether you wear a little makeup or a lot, there was probably a time in your life when you loved to experiment with it. Or maybe it's an ongoing give-and-take—you love your bold red lipstick today, but three months from now? Eh, not so much. And what about some of your past love affairs with makeup? Remember that short flirtation with turquoise mascara? Or when black nail polish had you smitten? Hey, we love a dark shade too!

There's no denying that makeup should be fun and uplifting, but that doesn't mean it can't also be practical and time efficient. That's where we come in. From the pages of *InStyle* magazine, we've gathered more than 200 tips from our editors, top-notch makeup pros, and Hollywood's biggest stars to help you find the colors and techniques that suit your style without sacrificing the fun. If you're a makeup novice or even if you've got the fundamentals under your belt, we guarantee you'll discover tons of new lip, cheek, eye, skin, and nail ideas and inspiration to add to your makeup bag of tricks. Get started now!

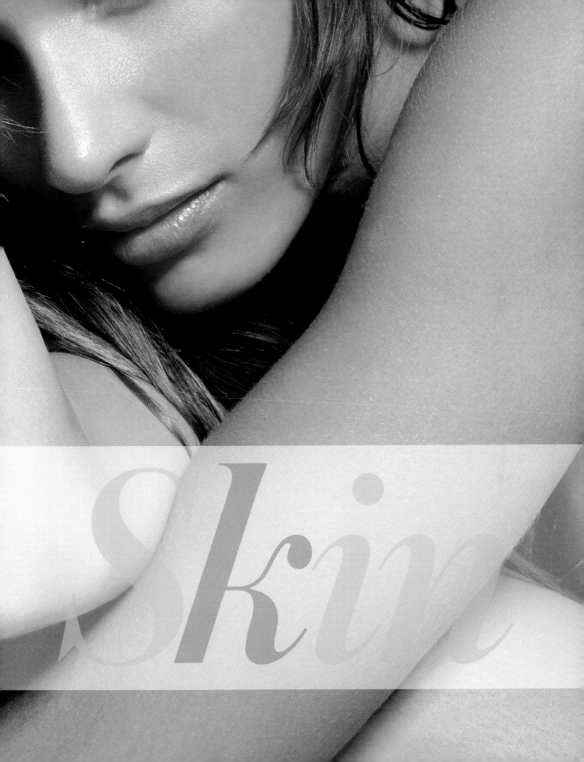

Skin

Traditional cleansers may not get skin 100 percent clean if you wear full-coverage foundation or SPF 45 (or higher) sunscreen. Instead, try A CLEANSING OIL. Massage it over dry skin to dissolve hard-to-remove products. Then use a REGULAR CLEANSER to wash your face.

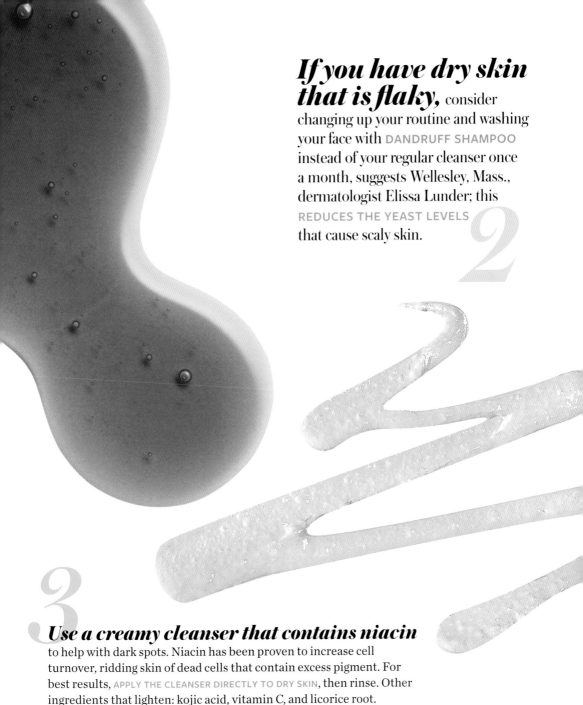

If you have dry skin that is flaky, consider changing up your routine and washing your face with DANDRUFF SHAMPOO instead of your regular cleanser once a month, suggests Wellesley, Mass., dermatologist Elissa Lunder; this REDUCES THE YEAST LEVELS that cause scaly skin.

Use a creamy cleanser that contains niacin

to help with dark spots. Niacin has been proven to increase cell turnover, ridding skin of dead cells that contain excess pigment. For best results, APPLY THE CLEANSER DIRECTLY TO DRY SKIN, then rinse. Other ingredients that lighten: kojic acid, vitamin C, and licorice root.

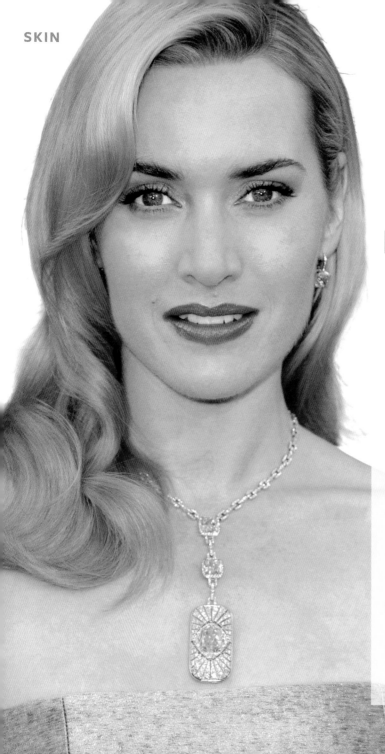

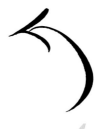

4

RED-CARPET SECRET

"A GOOD EYE CREAM IS REALLY IMPORTANT WHEN YOU'RE TRAVELING, BUSY AND STRESSED— THAT'S WHEN THE DARK, PUFFY CIRCLES CAN GET YOU."
—KATE WINSLET

5

{ *get rid of* *facial fuzz* }

Use gentle stripless waxes, which are made for smaller areas than strip waxes. Following the instructions on the box, test the wax on the inside of your wrist to make sure you have no adverse reaction. Then wipe the area to be waxed with rubbing alcohol to prevent breakouts and ingrown hairs. To apply, pull skin taut and spread on a banana-peel-thick layer in the direction of hair growth. Pull wax off in the opposite direction. Finish with a swipe of alcohol and some soothing oil. Be sure to exfoliate daily to prevent ingrown hairs. If you do see one, resist the temptation to pick at it. Instead, "use a 1 percent hydrocortisone cream to relieve redness and any itching or inflammation," says Ellen Marmur, chief of dermatologic and cosmetic surgery at Mount Sinai Medical Center in New York City. This should free the hair in about three days.

6

For stubborn eye makeup, first saturate a cotton square (it's less abrasive than a cotton ball) with an OIL-BASED REMOVER. Press over eyes for 30 seconds before gently wiping away, then rinse away oil completely with a regular cleanser. If you have dry skin, just WIPE AWAY EXCESS OIL with your cotton pad, allowing a bit to remain on skin to moisturize it.

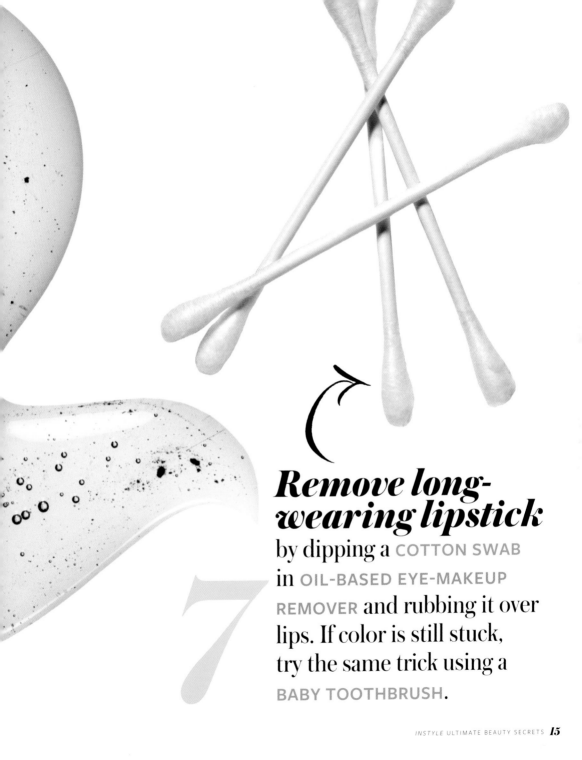

Remove long-wearing lipstick

by dipping a COTTON SWAB in OIL-BASED EYE-MAKEUP REMOVER and rubbing it over lips. If color is still stuck, try the same trick using a BABY TOOTHBRUSH.

7

8

Clean your cell phone with antibacterial wipes to prevent chin and cheek breakouts. Ideally, you should do it EVERY MORNING, but if that's too much, aim for once a week.

9

Use separate towels to dry your face and hair. This prevents the oils from your scalp from rubbing off on your face and CAUSING BREAKOUTS.

10

To rid makeup brushes of products that can clog pores, aim to wash them with a CLARIFYING SHAMPOO once a week.

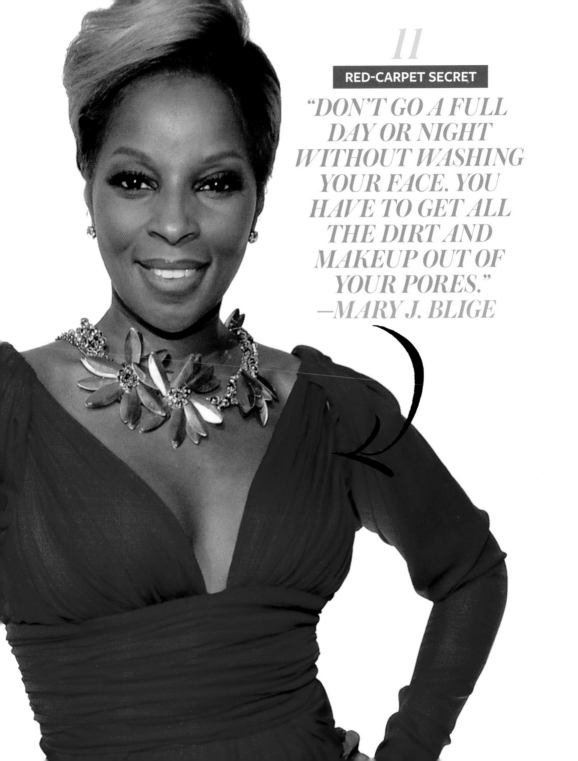

11

"DON'T GO A FULL DAY OR NIGHT WITHOUT WASHING YOUR FACE. YOU HAVE TO GET ALL THE DIRT AND MAKEUP OUT OF YOUR PORES."
—MARY J. BLIGE

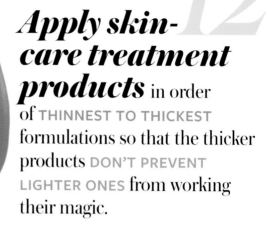

Apply skin-care treatment products in order of THINNEST TO THICKEST formulations so that the thicker products DON'T PREVENT LIGHTER ONES from working their magic.

12

13

A single piece of tissue can help you figure out your skin type. Wash and dry your face and leave it unmoisturized for three hours. Then PRESS A TISSUE TO YOUR FACE AND REMOVE IT. You have NORMAL skin if no oil comes off on the tissue and your face doesn't feel tight or flaky. You have DRY skin if no oil comes off but your face feels dry, tight or flaky. You have OILY skin if there's oil from your nose, forehead and cheeks. You have COMBINATION skin if there's oil from your nose and forehead (the areas of the face with the most oil glands) but not your cheeks. Pick skin-care products that are formulated for your skin type.

The day before a party, don't risk a facial that can leave you red and raw. An *at-home mask* made with one teaspoon raw oatmeal and one teaspoon honey is a much safer bet. Let it sit on skin for five minutes, then rinse. "The minerals in oatmeal are soothing, and *honey hydrates* and kills bacteria," says aesthetician Kate Somerville, who has worked with *Kate Walsh* and *Debra Messing*.

15

New skin-care regimens take time to work. Allow six weeks to three months

for ACNE-FIGHTERS TO TAKE EFFECT, six to 12 months for a SKIN-LIGHTENING regimen, and three months for an ANTI-AGING ROUTINE. One caveat: If you develop a rash, swelling, redness, or itching, you may be allergic to the product or applying it incorrectly. Stop using it immediately and consult your doctor.

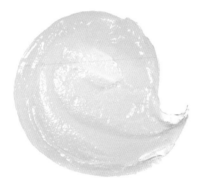

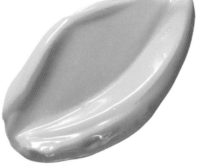

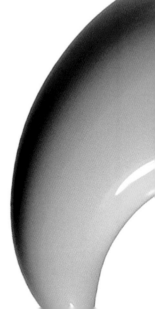

16

After cleansing and before layering on sunscreen, use an

ANTIOXIDANT SERUM to clear out free radicals and help prevent wrinkles from forming, suggests Washington, D.C., dermatologist Tina Alster. Bonus: The serum also makes YOUR SPF MORE EFFECTIVE.

17

If retinoids make your skin too dry, try using

them AT NIGHT, when your oil production surges. Formulas with soothing vitamin E and green tea also help MINIMIZE DRYNESS.

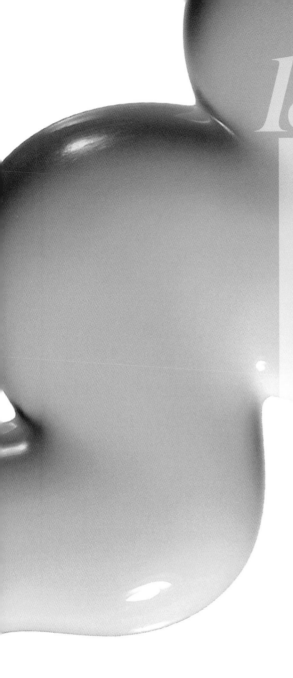

18

{ *fight wrinkles* } *in 3 steps*

1. Use an exfoliating alpha-hydroxy cleanser in the morning, then a serum with hyaluronic acid, which has a plumping effect, to fill in lines, suggests N.Y.C. dermatologist Howard Sobel.

2. Next, shield skin from the sun (alpha-hydroxys make skin extra photosensitive) and use antioxidants to neutralize the free radicals that contribute to aging. Apply an antioxidant day cream with an SPF of 30 or higher.

3. At night, focus on repair, says Miami Beach dermatologist Leslie Baumann. Use your morning cleanser, then an anti-aging night cream with retinol to stimulate collagen production.

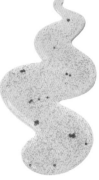

19 *Sensitive skin often can't take too many active ingredients.* So after using a FRAGRANCE-FREE CLEANSER, moisturize with a serum that has anti-inflammatory antioxidants such as green tea.

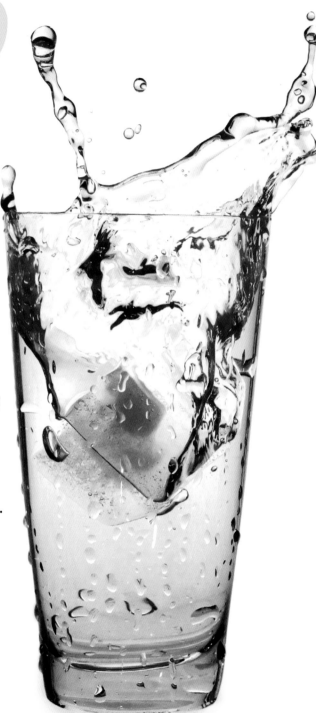

20 *Drink a glass of ice water if your face tends to get splotchy* (especially when you're nervous). Doing so will TONE DOWN YOUR REDNESS. The cold causes blood vessels to constrict and COOL YOU from the inside out, says dermatologist Ellen Marmur.

21

{ Summer
Skin
Trick }

When the temps rise, layer your moisturizer to *fight dryness* caused by sun, heat, chlorine, and salt water. Use a hydrating wash in the shower (look for one with vitamins B3 and B5 to help reduce water loss), then apply a *light lotion* to further soften skin, suggests N.Y.C. dermatologist Lisa Airan.

22

To control oil and shine, splash your face with COOL BLACK TEA, but do not rinse; it's A NATURAL ASTRINGENT, says Beverly Hills dermatologist Peter Kopelson.

23

Refresh your complexion by dipping a washcloth in soy milk and resting it on your face for 10 minutes once a week, suggests Beverly Hills dermatologist Debra Luftman. SOY IS A SKIN BRIGHTENER and contains phytoestrogen, a plant-derived estrogen that is thought to help PREVENT WRINKLES.

RED-CARPET SECRET

"I USE OMEGA-3 OIL. I LOVE LIGHT OIL ON MY SKIN. IT'S ONE OF MY FAVORITE FEELINGS IN THE WORLD." —GWYNETH PALTROW

25

Reduce a pimple's redness by spritzing a small amount of NASAL DECONGESTANT on the blemish, says Mount Kisco, N.Y., dermatologist David Bank. The spray, designed to LESSEN INFLAMMATION, will do the same for a pimple.

26

To get rid of blackheads, use a low-dose 5 percent benzoyl peroxide solution to kill bacteria and break down and remove dead cells. Then EXFOLIATE with a salicylic acid buffing pad to gently POLISH THE SKIN.

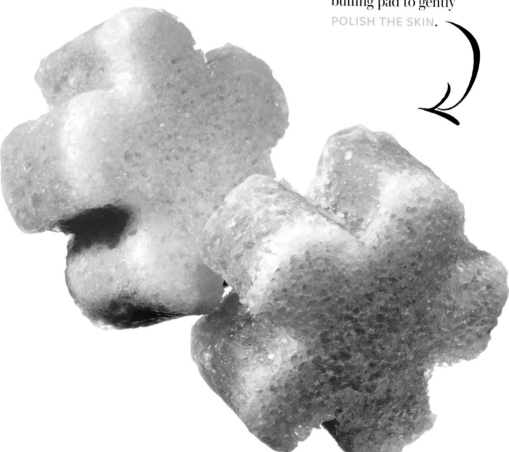

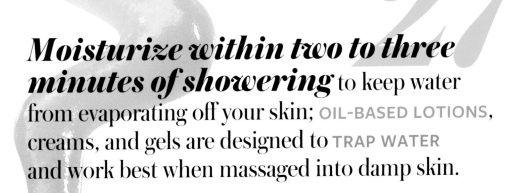

27

Moisturize within two to three minutes of showering to keep water from evaporating off your skin; OIL-BASED LOTIONS, creams, and gels are designed to TRAP WATER and work best when massaged into damp skin.

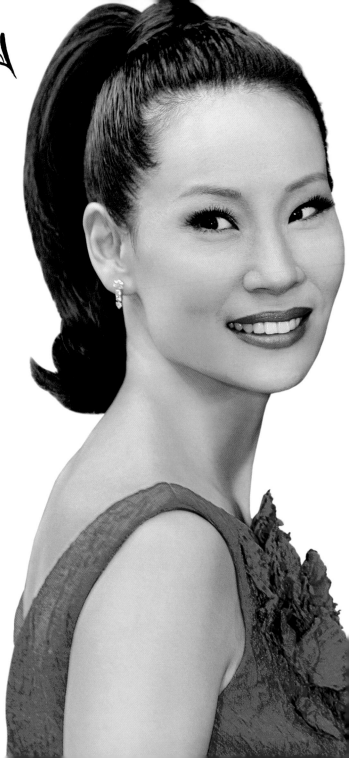

28

"WHEN I WAS SHOOTING A MOVIE IN MONTREAL, IT WAS FREEZING. IF YOU TAKE A LITTLE BIT OF AQUAPHOR AND DAB IT ON YOUR FACE, IT KEEPS YOUR SKIN LOOKING FRESH. I DUBBED IT AQUA FOR EVERYTHING."
—LUCY LIU

29

Get the most out of your moisturizer by switching formulations from day to night. "Sunscreen is probably taking the place of another THERAPEUTIC INGREDIENT," explains N.Y.C. dermatologist Patricia Wexler, who has worked with Iman. So use a moisturizer with sunscreen DURING THE DAY, and one with other active ingredients, like retinol, AT NIGHT.

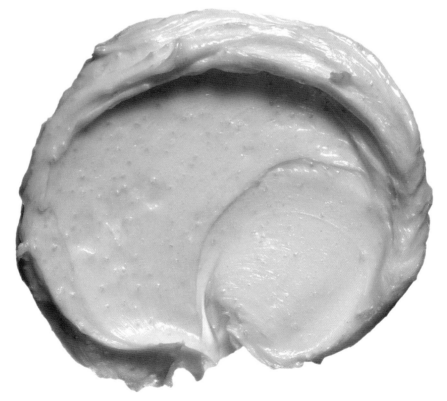

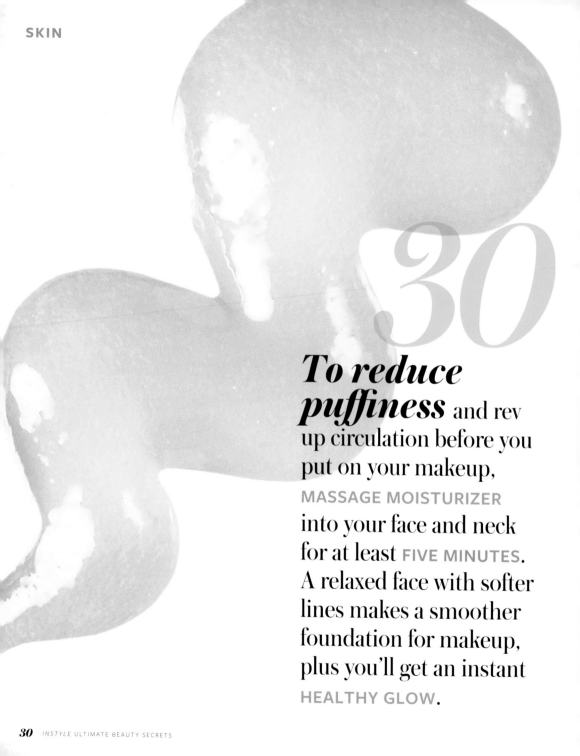

30

To reduce puffiness and rev up circulation before you put on your makeup, MASSAGE MOISTURIZER into your face and neck for at least FIVE MINUTES. A relaxed face with softer lines makes a smoother foundation for makeup, plus you'll get an instant HEALTHY GLOW.

Keep skin hydrated on cold nights with a *make-it-yourself humidifier*. Meriden, Conn., dermatologist Nicholas V. Perricone suggests hanging *a wet towel* from the doorknob overnight (wring out the edges to prevent drips); by morning, the towel will be dry but your skin won't.

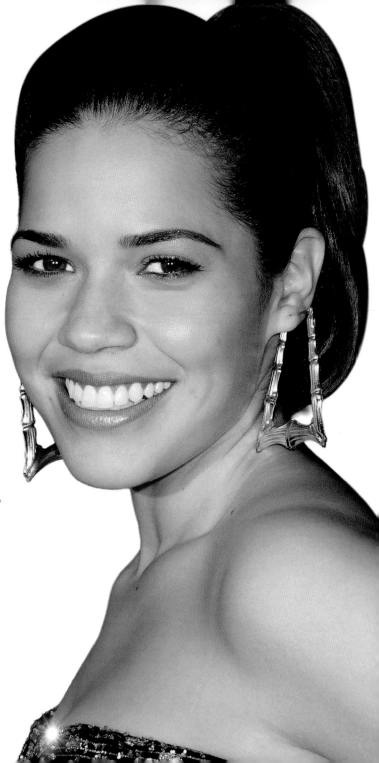

32

"ONCE I STARTED DRINKING MORE WATER, MY SKIN, HAIR AND NAILS ALL FLOURISHED." —AMERICA FERRERA

33

It takes 30 minutes for sunscreen to absorb fully into your skin, so put it on before going outside and REAPPLY EVERY TWO HOURS; perspiration, heat, and swimming can diminish the SPF's efficacy.

34

Consider using a different SPF cream on your neck than on your face, says Bruce Katz, director, Juva Skin and Laser Center in N.Y.C. "For some people, skin on the neck, which tends to be more sensitive than facial skin, may become red and irritated with the use of CHEMICAL SUNSCREEN," he warns. "In that case, try a physical block with ZINC OXIDE OR TITANIUM DIOXIDE."

35

If sunscreen irritates the thin, delicate skin around your eyes,

it may be that the chemicals are causing A REACTION. Try a MINERAL FORMULA or gentle baby sunscreen instead.

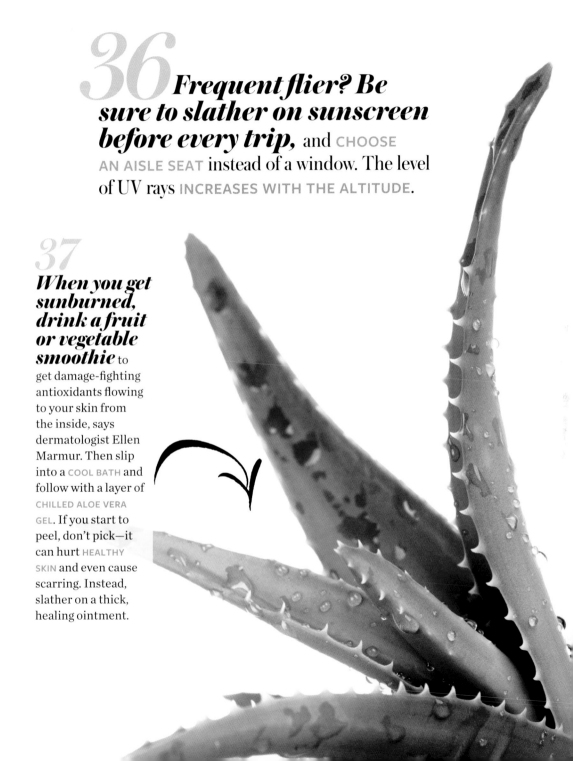

36 *Frequent flier? Be sure to slather on sunscreen before every trip,* and CHOOSE AN AISLE SEAT instead of a window. The level of UV rays INCREASES WITH THE ALTITUDE.

37

When you get sunburned, drink a fruit or vegetable smoothie to get damage-fighting antioxidants flowing to your skin from the inside, says dermatologist Ellen Marmur. Then slip into a COOL BATH and follow with a layer of CHILLED ALOE VERA GEL. If you start to peel, don't pick—it can hurt HEALTHY SKIN and even cause scarring. Instead, slather on a thick, healing ointment.

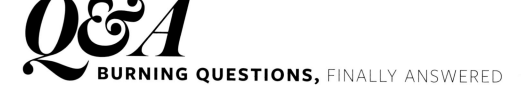

Q&A
BURNING QUESTIONS, FINALLY ANSWERED

IN THE SUMMER, I GET DARK PATCHES ON MY SKIN THAT I THINK ARE SUN SPOTS, BUT I'VE ALSO HEARD ABOUT A SKIN CONDITION CALLED MELASMA. WHAT'S THE DIFFERENCE?

Sun spots are small brown spots on any part of the body caused by overactive pigment production as a result of sun exposure; they may be as small as a piece of confetti or as large as a dime. Melasma patches occur only on the face and can be as large as a quarter; they are more common in women with darker skin. Melasma is usually triggered by changes in estrogen levels (from pregnancy or birth control pills) in combination with sun exposure. If you think you have melasma, avoid the sun and wear a broad-spectrum sunblock of SPF 30 or higher to prevent the patches from getting darker.

IS THERE ANY WAY TO PREVENT A SCAR FROM FORMING—OR TO MAKE ONE GO AWAY?

Keeping a wound moist and clean can minimize the chance of scarring. Immediately, and once a day after the injury, gently wash your wound with warm, soapy water; rinse, and apply an antibiotic ointment such as Neosporin. Then cover the wound with a bandage. If you do scar, there's no way to make it totally vanish, but you can minimize its appearance. Since scars are at risk for hyperpigmentation, always cover them with sunscreen when out in the sun. To lighten scars, try hydroquinone cream. Red scars can be treated with a laser by your dermatologist. And if you develop a keloid scar, which has a thick, raised surface, give it a daily 20-minute fingertip massage; the repeated pressure can help break up the fibrous bands. You can also ask your dermatologist about cortisone injections, which will help dissolve the built-up scar tissue.

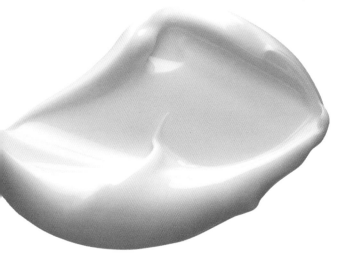

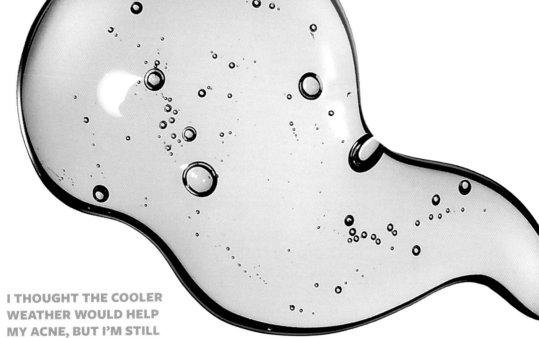

I THOUGHT THE COOLER WEATHER WOULD HELP MY ACNE, BUT I'M STILL BREAKING OUT. WHAT'S THE PROBLEM?

Cold weather slows the skin's natural exfoliation process, which can exacerbate breakouts, explains N.Y.C. dermatologist Dennis Gross. The key is to slough off dead skin cells daily before they have a chance to clog pores. Gross recommends using a mild astringent cleanser containing witch hazel (which also functions as an anti-irritant), plus an oil-free moisturizer that has broad-spectrum sun protection. For night, he suggests a gentle peel before bed, explaining, "The skin secretes oil while you sleep, which will counteract any dryness caused by the peel."

I'D LIKE TO USE RETINOL PRODUCTS, BUT I HAVE SENSITIVE SKIN. WHAT CAN I DO TO PREVENT IRRITATION?

Regardless of your skin type, you have to slowly build up tolerance when using this potent vitamin A derivative to treat fine lines. "Retinol can be very drying," explains N.Y.C. dermatologist Anne Chapas, assistant clinical professor at New York University School of Medicine. Apply just a pea-size amount divided over the four quadrants of the face (right and left cheeks, chin and forehead) every other night for the first week. Gradually increase application (two nights on, one night off) until you can tolerate it every night. But note: Some women may never be able to use retinol products every night.

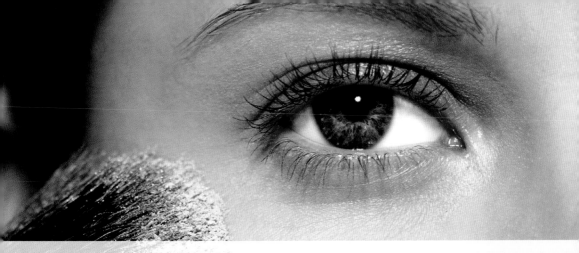
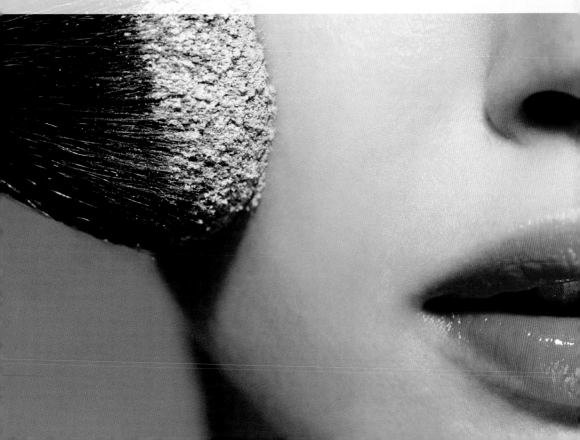

Foundation & Concealer

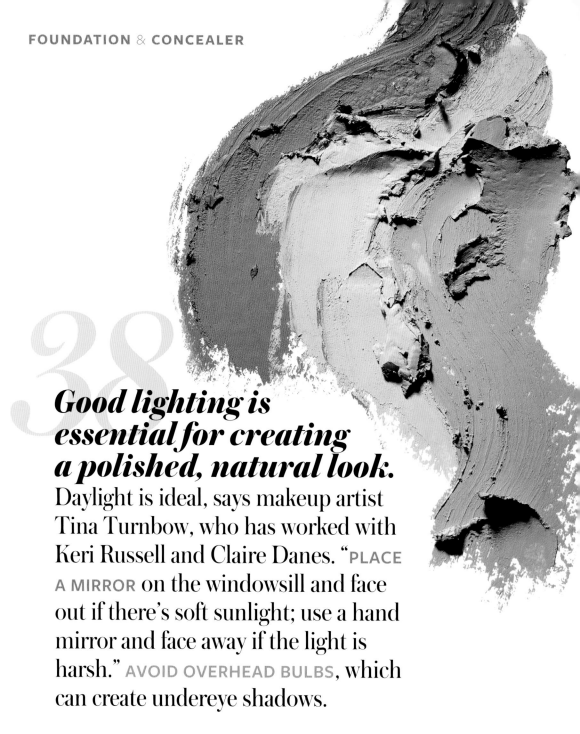

38

Good lighting is essential for creating a polished, natural look.

Daylight is ideal, says makeup artist Tina Turnbow, who has worked with Keri Russell and Claire Danes. "PLACE A MIRROR on the windowsill and face out if there's soft sunlight; use a hand mirror and face away if the light is harsh." AVOID OVERHEAD BULBS, which can create undereye shadows.

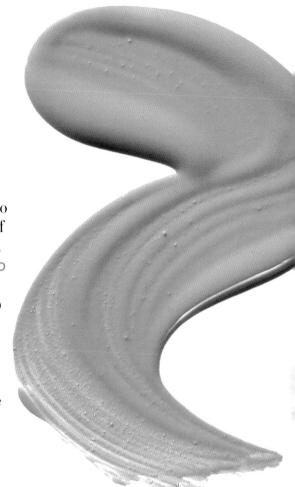

39

Test colors on your jawline and throat—not

your face, wrist, or hand—says makeup artist Mally Roncal, who has helped perfect the visages of stars like Rihanna and Beyoncé. "The right one will VANISH INTO YOUR SKIN." Always check the color in daylight; at the makeup counter, ask for a hand mirror to take outside. Shop for one shade in SUMMER (when skin is generally darker) and another one in WINTER. Then blend the two for transitional seasons.

40

For extra-natural-looking skin,

try a TINTED MOISTURIZER. Since it's LIGHTWEIGHT, it won't cover dark spots, blemishes, or red blotches, but it will EVEN OUT SKIN TONE.

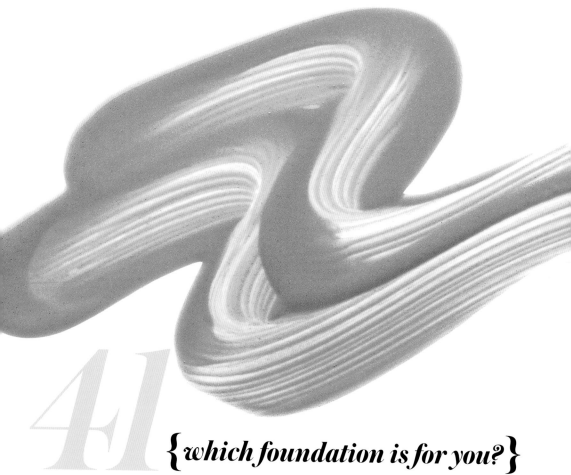

41

{ *which foundation is for you?* }

Oil-free liquid foundation produces a natural "no-makeup" look on oily skin. If your skin is super-shiny, an oil-absorbing powder is a great way to give your face a matte finish.

If you have combination skin, look for foundation that's billed as "balancing," since those are specifically formulated for skin that's both dry and oily.

"Hydrating" or "moisture-rich" foundations are best for dry skin, since these products have moisturizing ingredients and skin-softeners such as vitamin E, hyaluronic acid, and glycerin.

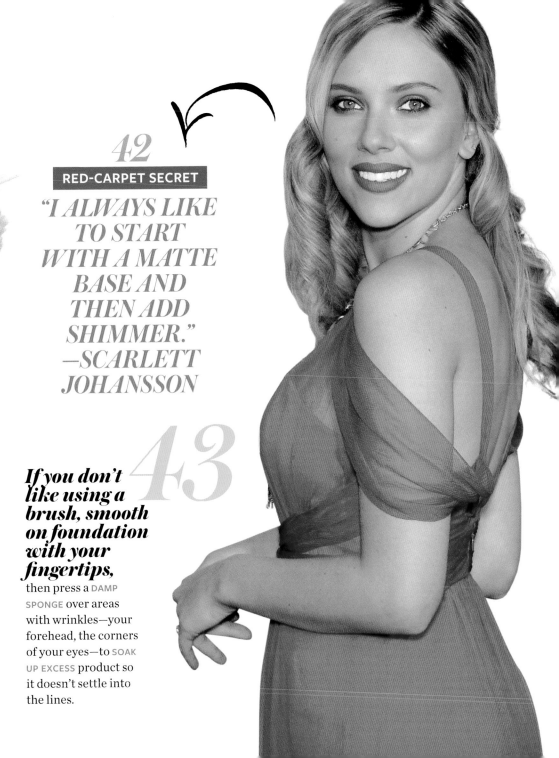

42

"I ALWAYS LIKE TO START WITH A MATTE BASE AND THEN ADD SHIMMER."
—SCARLETT JOHANSSON

43

If you don't like using a brush, smooth on foundation with your fingertips, then press a DAMP SPONGE over areas with wrinkles—your forehead, the corners of your eyes—to SOAK UP EXCESS product so it doesn't settle into the lines.

44

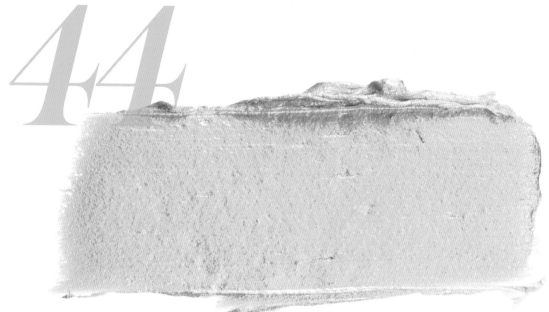

Many women need to use two shades of foundation to create the PERFECT MATCH—a darker shade around the sides of the face, and a slightly lighter one on the cheekbones and the nose to CATCH THE LIGHT.

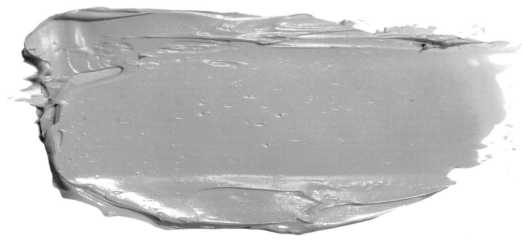

{ Summer Foundation Trick }

Foundation can reduce redness caused by a sunburn. Choose a *golden shade* with warm undertones to turn the burn into a *glow*. Just don't choose a hue lighter than your *natural skin* tone or the overall effect will look ghostly.

46

If your skin has red undertones, choose a foundation with some yellow (or even green) tones to NEUTRALIZE YOUR COMPLEXION.

For sun protection, use a foundation with SPF or apply a moisturizer that has SPF in it before you apply a non-SPF foundation. The LAYER OF MOISTURIZER will help foundation go on smoothly, and the SPF PROTECTS SKIN.

47

To make summer foundation work in winter, dab a *little foundation* on your hand, then squeeze a pea-size blob of *SPF 30* on top and mix until the sunscreen blends completely with the foundation, lightening it by a shade or two.

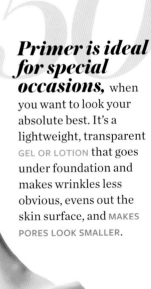

49

To keep liquid foundation from fading, mix it with a drop of SWEAT-PROOF SUNBLOCK, then smooth it on. It will last all night, even if you dance up a storm.

50

Primer is ideal for special occasions, when you want to look your absolute best. It's a lightweight, transparent GEL OR LOTION that goes under foundation and makes wrinkles less obvious, evens out the skin surface, and MAKES PORES LOOK SMALLER.

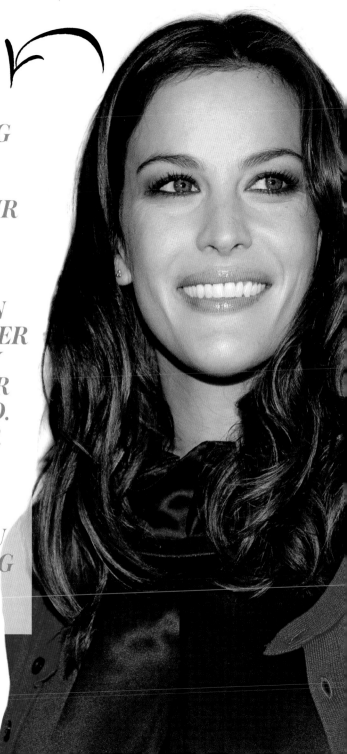

51

"AFTER APPLYING FOUNDATION AND A LITTLE BLUSH, DUST YOUR FACE WITH TRANSLUCENT POWDER, THEN MIST SKIN WITH A ROSEWATER SPRAY AND LAY A KLEENEX OVER IT FOR A SECOND. IT MAKES YOUR FACE SEEM FLAWLESS IN A WAY THAT LOOKS AS IF YOU AREN'T WEARING MAKEUP."
—LIV TYLER

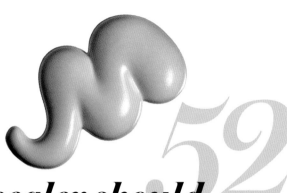

Concealer should always follow foundation;

52

if you put it on first and *then* BLEND FOUNDATION, the foundation will cover up the concealer.

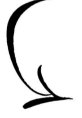

Cover up undereye circles with a light, creamy concealer by using a SMALL, FIRM-BRISTLE brush. Or dab it on with your ring finger, which won't apply as much pressure as your index finger, so you DON'T TUG ON DELICATE EYE SKIN. Just be sure to pat—not rub—it in.

53

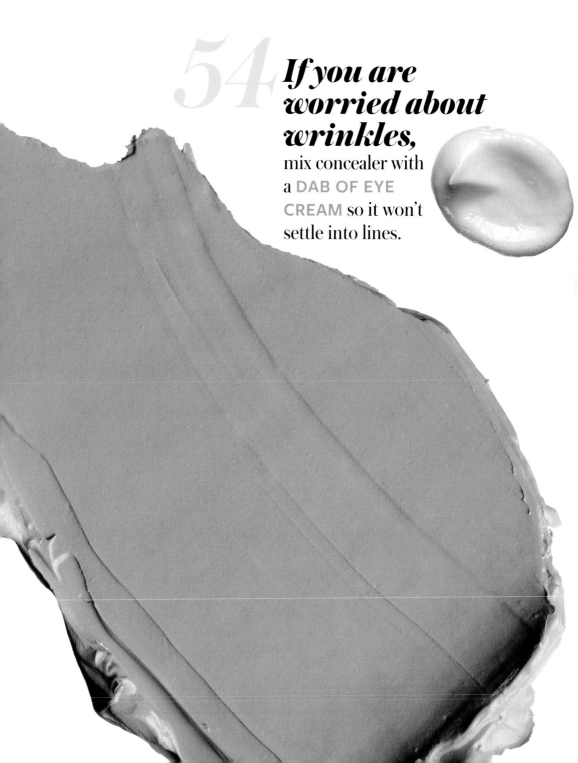

54

If you are worried about wrinkles, mix concealer with a DAB OF EYE CREAM so it won't settle into lines.

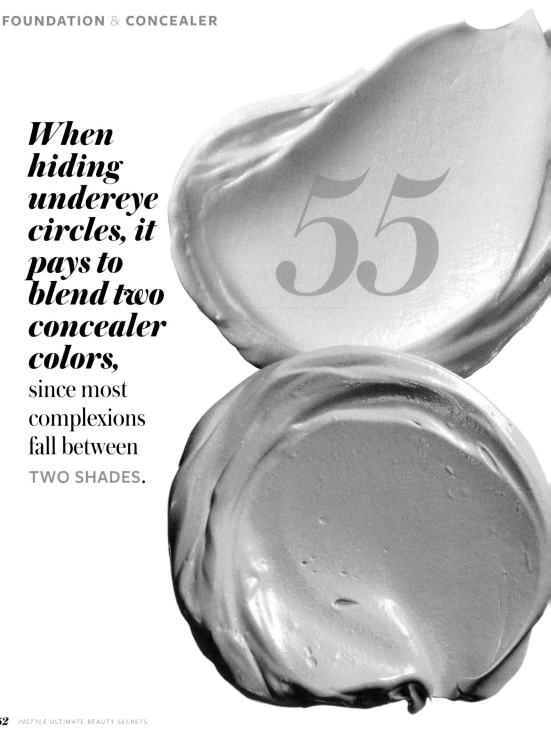

When hiding undereye circles, it pays to blend two concealer colors, since most complexions fall between TWO SHADES.

55

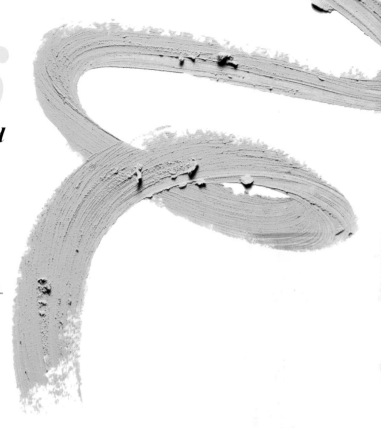

56

If you need to hide a blemish, pick an oil-free concealer that has SALICYLIC ACID, BENZOYL PEROXIDE, or SULFUR to treat while you conceal.

57

Use a clean eyeliner brush to apply concealer over blemishes. It's smaller than a standard concealer brush, so the product winds up ONLY ON THE BLEMISH, not the surrounding skin.

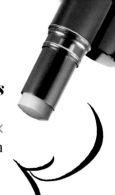

58 Liquid concealers can be too sheer

when COVERING UP DARK SPOTS, so opt for a cream or stick formula.

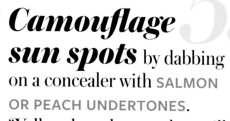

Camouflage 59 sun spots by dabbing

on a concealer with SALMON OR PEACH UNDERTONES. "Yellow-based concealers will cause the spot to look gray," warns celebrity makeup artist Lauren Kaye Cohen.

A yellow-tinted neutralizing concealer balances out red blotches.

If color peeks through, use your fingertip to dab a more OPAQUE YELLOW-TONED CONCEALER just on those areas.

60

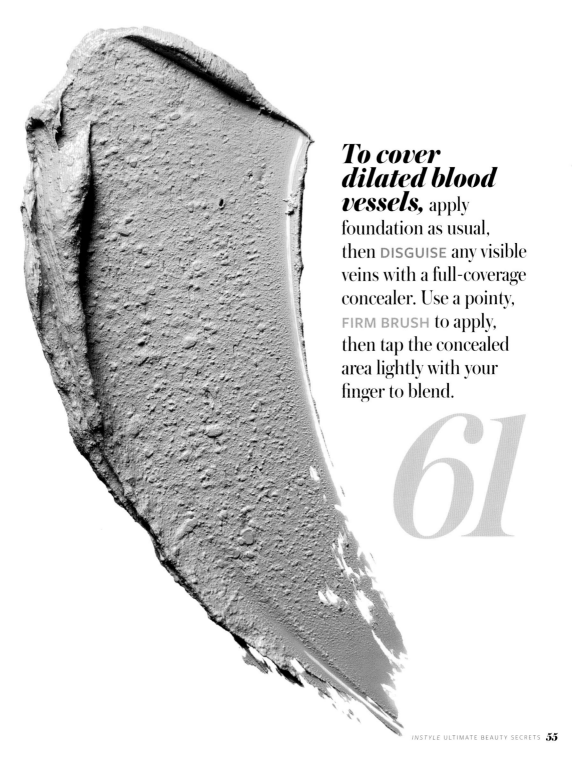

To cover dilatd blood vessels, apply foundation as usual, then DISGUISE any visible veins with a full-coverage concealer. Use a pointy, FIRM BRUSH to apply, then tap the concealed area lightly with your finger to blend.

61

Q&A

BURNING QUESTIONS, FINALLY ANSWERED

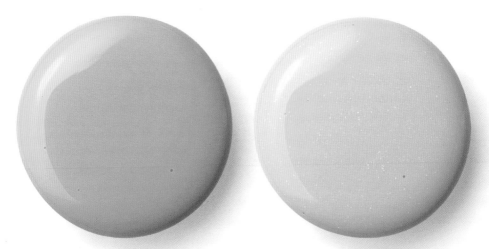

WHY DOES IT LOOK AS IF I HAVE WHITISH RINGS UNDER MY EYES IN PHOTOS?

Your concealer is too light. Even if you're sure you bought the right color, daily sun can slightly darken your skin. This is why celebrity makeup artist Laura Mercier, who has worked with Sarah Jessica Parker, Julia Roberts, and Juliette Binoche, swears by duo concealer compacts. "One shade should match your lightest skin tone, and the second your darkest," she says. Blending the two works for your "in-between" phases. Set with a light dusting of translucent powder.

I'M AFRAID THAT MY SKIN WILL GET SHINY WHEN I DANCE ALL NIGHT. HOW CAN I AVOID IT?

Prepare skin with a mattifying primer. When you put it on your T-zone, you can literally watch it soak up the oils, says N.Y.C. makeup artist Mario Dedivanovic, who has worked with Kim Kardashian. "The primer won't block sweat, but it will absorb it and create a barrier between your skin and the rest of your makeup." If too much boogying still leaves you glistening like a disco ball, simply wick away sweat with blotting papers.

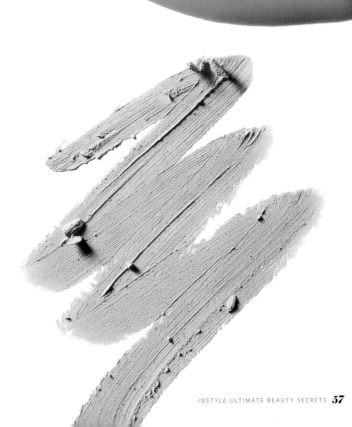

WHAT SHOULD I DO IF I'VE PUT ON TOO MUCH FOUNDATION?

With clean hands, lightly sweep both palms in smooth motions over your face to soak up excess makeup. Don't rub or pull at your skin; you'll wipe off sections of base and be forced to start over from scratch. If sweeping doesn't do the trick, press (but don't rub) a piece of tissue over your face to absorb excess product, and be sure to soften lines of demarcation between your face and neck with a damp makeup sponge.

CAN I USE FOUNDATION AS CONCEALER?

If you don't have a lot to cover and you really want the convenience of using just one product, a dense, full-bodied foundation might do the job. But most foundations are thinner in texture and tend to move around a bit, so they don't give the precise coverage you'd get from a thicker, more deeply pigmented concealer. In a pinch, you can use the densely packed foundation accumulated in the opening of the bottle to cover up imperfections. But if you have relatively clear skin, you're better off skipping the foundation altogether and just tackling trouble spots with the right concealer.

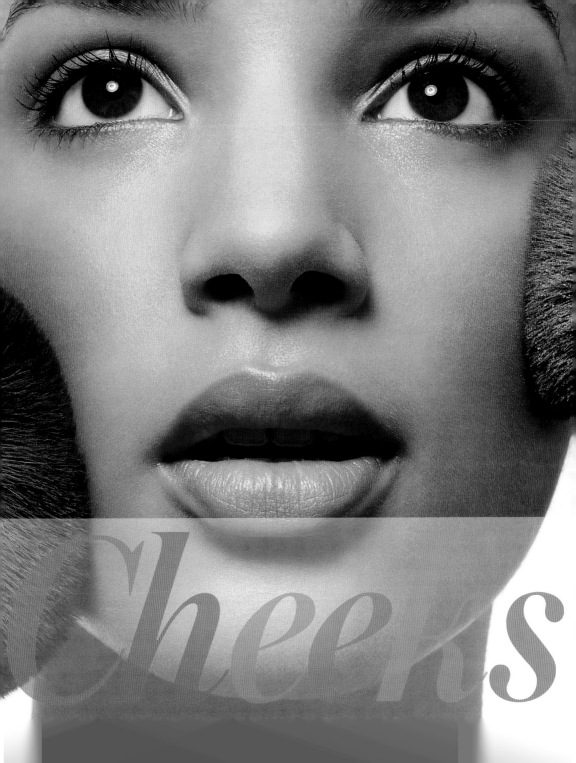

Cheeks

62

Powder blushes work on all skin types, but are ideal for OILY SKIN and should be applied with a big, fluffy brush. BONUS: They are long lasting.

63

Cream blushes are best on dry or aging skin because of their rich, MOISTURIZING PROPERTIES; they are tougher to use on oily skin because they don't blend as well.

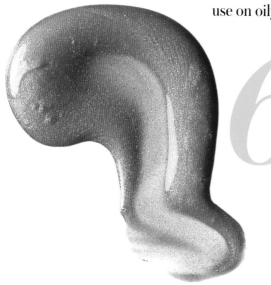

64

Fast-drying gel and liquid blushes and cheek stains have super staying power and work well on normal to oily skin, but they can be HARD TO SPREAD ONTO DRY SKIN. Since you apply them with your fingertips, you have to wash your hands immediately afterward to avoid staining fingers.

Powder blush doesn't handle sweat well. When the weather heats up, choose a *cream blush* or *liquid cheek stain* instead.

CHEEKS

66

WARM

Pick cheek colors that complement your skin tone. WARM COMPLEXIONS look best in yellow-based blush shades like peach and terracotta; COOL UNDERTONES are flattered by blue-based pinks and berries. Not sure if you are warm or cool complected? FIND YOUR PERFECT CHEEK COLOR THIS WAY: At the hardware store, pick up paint chips in colors that you think could work as blush. Hold the chips up to your face in front of a mirror in natural light; you'll instantly see WHAT BRIGHTENS YOUR COMPLEXION vs. what makes it look sallow or gray.

COOL

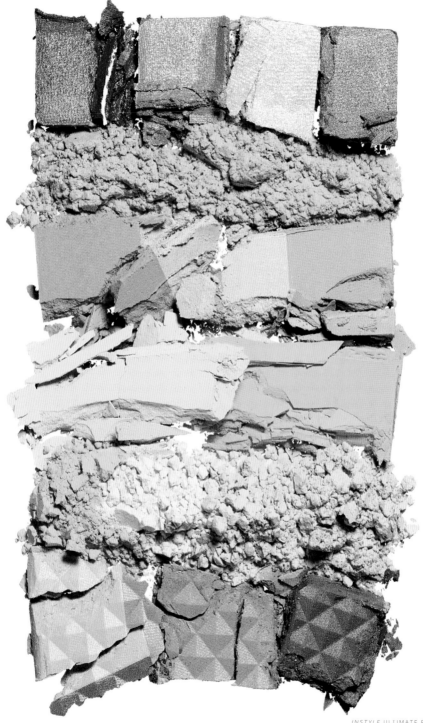

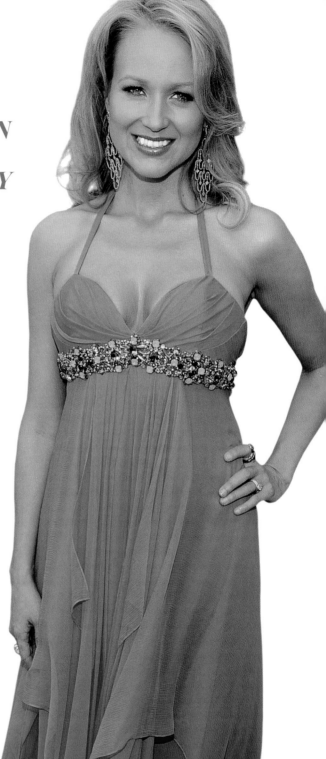

67

"I WEAR LIP STAIN ON MY CHEEKS UNDERNEATH MY FOUNDATION."
—JEWEL

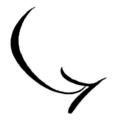

68

Lighter blush shades roll back the clock, says makeup artist Troy Surratt, who has worked with CHARLIZE THERON and CARRIE UNDERWOOD. "Let your cheeks glow subtly with a rosy or peach-tone blush."

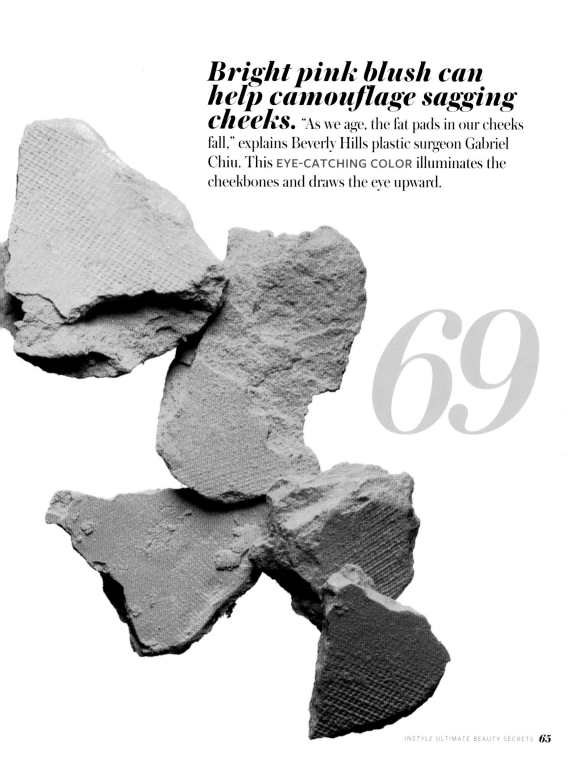

Bright pink blush can help camouflage sagging cheeks.

"As we age, the fat pads in our cheeks fall," explains Beverly Hills plastic surgeon Gabriel Chiu. This EYE-CATCHING COLOR illuminates the cheekbones and draws the eye upward.

69

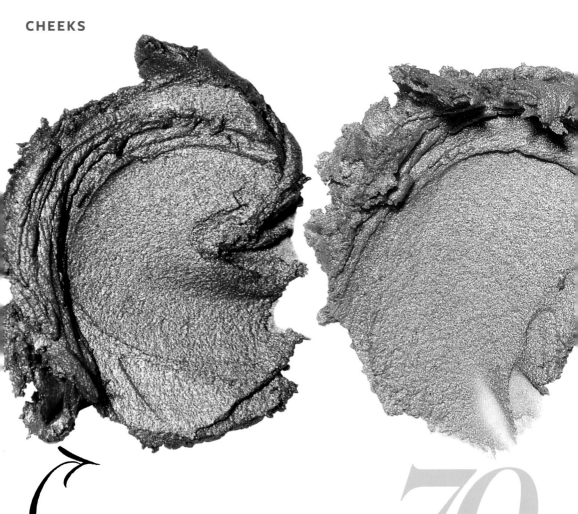

70

For the most natural look,

makeup artist Bobbi Brown suggests using TWO COLORS: one bronzy shade and one with a dash of color (brighter pink, coral, rose, or plum). Swirl the rosy hue on the apples, then blend a SWOOSH OF BRONZE below the cheekbones for definition.

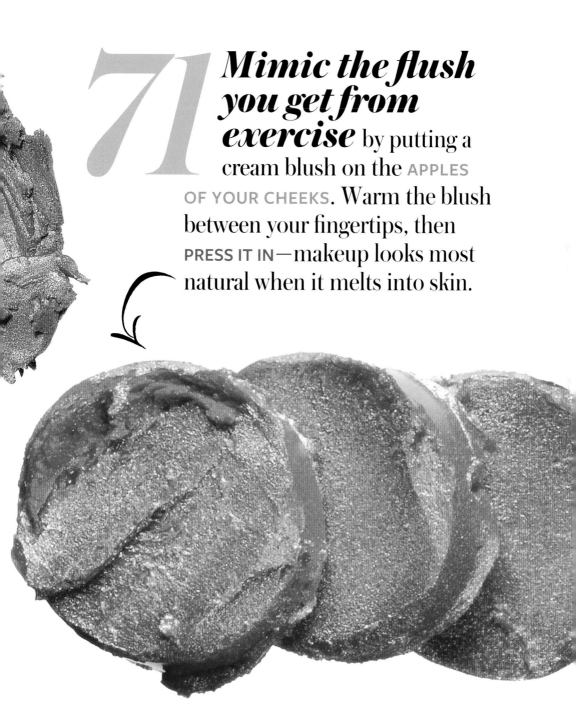

71

Mimic the flush you get from exercise by putting a cream blush on the APPLES OF YOUR CHEEKS. Warm the blush between your fingertips, then PRESS IT IN—makeup looks most natural when it melts into skin.

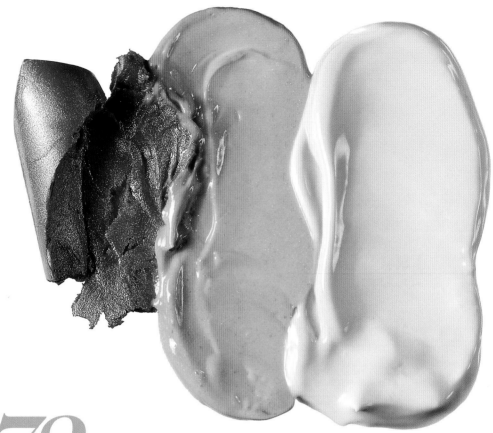

72 {*GENIUS IDEA!*}

Need a long-lasting blush in a pinch? Just rub your finger over a long-wearing lipstick three or four times, then, with a clean finger, take a swipe of your moisturizer. Mix the two together, then dot on cheeks and blend. You can also warm up long-lasting lip color on the back of your hand, then pat it onto your cheeks—just wash your hands quickly with an oil-based makeup remover to avoid staining.

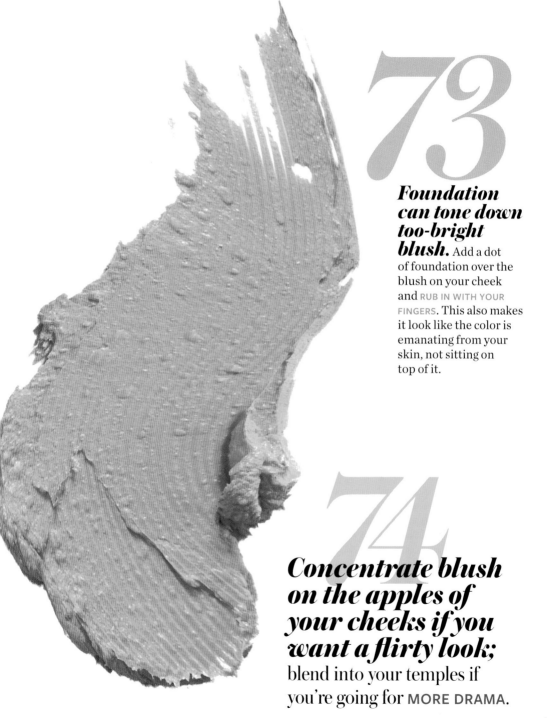

73

Foundation can tone down too-bright blush. Add a dot of foundation over the blush on your cheek and RUB IN WITH YOUR FINGERS. This also makes it look like the color is emanating from your skin, not sitting on top of it.

74

Concentrate blush on the apples of your cheeks if you want a flirty look; blend into your temples if you're going for MORE DRAMA.

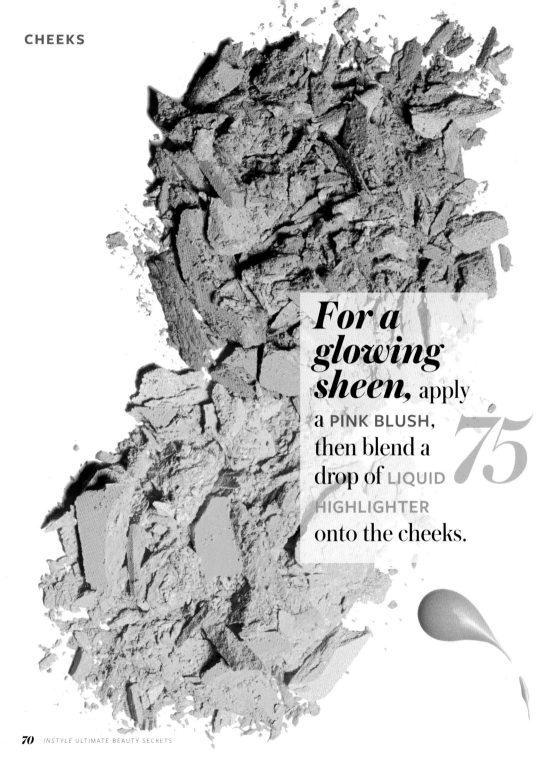

For a glowing sheen, apply a PINK BLUSH, then blend a drop of LIQUID HIGHLIGHTER onto the cheeks.

75

76

Make cheek color last longer by CHOOSING A BLUSH that's the SAME TEXTURE AS YOUR FOUNDATION— liquid on liquid, cream on cream, or powder on powder.

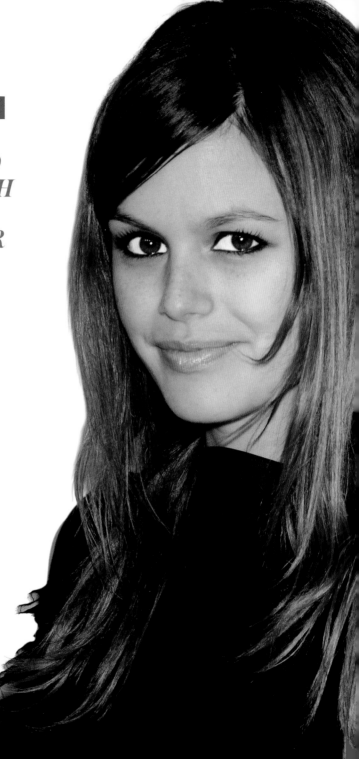

77

"I DUST MY CHEEKS AND EYELIDS WITH BRONZING POWDER FOR A NATURAL GLOW."
—RACHEL BILSON

78

Make sure cream blush stays on all day by using a primer. If you don't wear foundation, you can use PRIMER ALONE, smoothing it on just under the area where the cream blush is applied, or SPREADING IT OVER THE ENTIRE CHEEK. Either way, the primer will help set the cream blush.

79 *For the most authentic sun-kissed look,* apply bronzer where SUNLIGHT NATURALLY HITS— the center of your forehead, your cheekbones, and chin.

80 *If you want to achieve a light, all-over glow,* mix a touch of LIQUID BRONZER with your sunscreen.

81

For normal to oily complexions, apply powder bronzer with a short, fluffy brush, suggests makeup guru Bobbi Brown. CREAM BRONZER, applied with fingers or a sponge, is ideal for dry skin.

82

If you like bronzers that are shimmery, don't go extra dark. With shimmery pigments, "when you go too dark, it tends to LOOK DIRTY," warns Angela Levin, Jennifer Aniston's makeup artist.

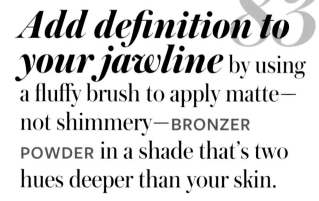

83

Add definition to your jawline by using a fluffy brush to apply matte—not shimmery—BRONZER POWDER in a shade that's two hues deeper than your skin.

Bronzer isn't just for the summer; in the winter it can make for a great evening look. Start with a loose, *rosy-brown powder* and concentrate color on cheekbones, then lightly dust your forehead, cheeks, and chin. Complete the look by adding a *shimmery peach blush* to the apples of cheeks.

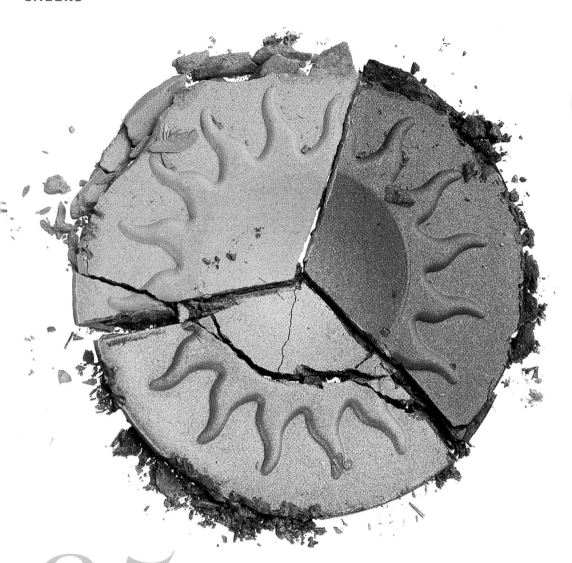

85

Be careful where you apply powder bronzer. "No powder around laugh lines, nose, or eyes; it adds darkness and ages you," warns JENNIFER LOPEZ's makeup artist, Scott Barnes.

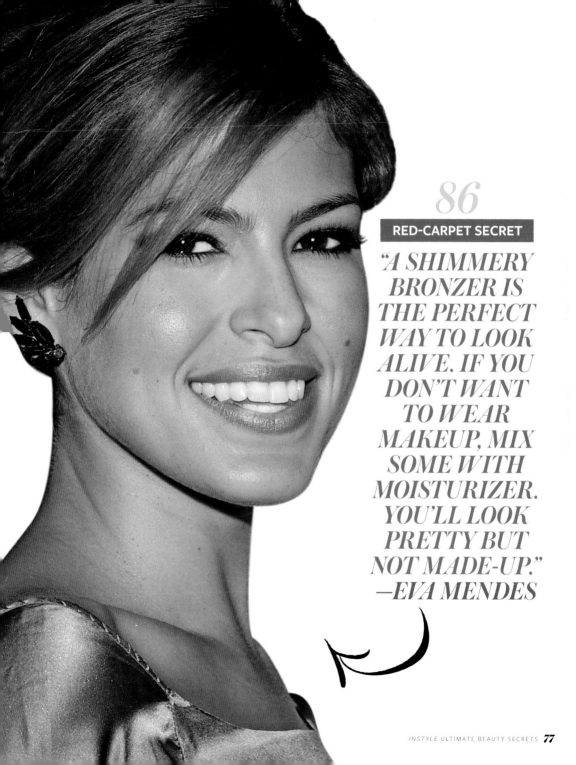

86

"A SHIMMERY BRONZER IS THE PERFECT WAY TO LOOK ALIVE. IF YOU DON'T WANT TO WEAR MAKEUP, MIX SOME WITH MOISTURIZER. YOU'LL LOOK PRETTY BUT NOT MADE-UP."
—EVA MENDES

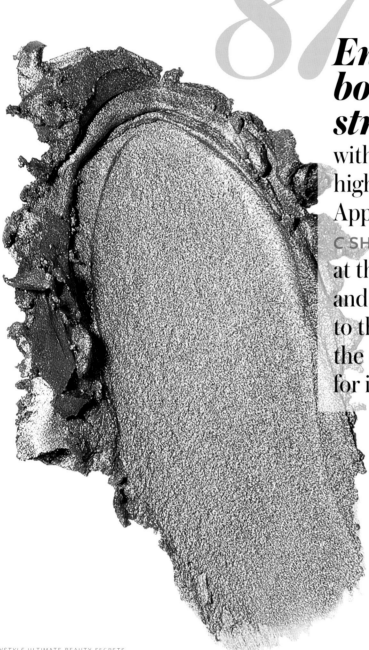

87

Enhance bone structure

with luminizing highlighter. Apply it in a C SHAPE, starting at the temples and extending out to the tops of the cheekbones for impact.

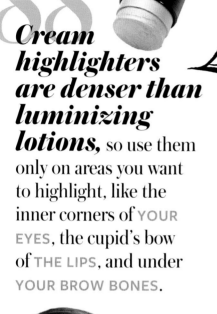

88

Cream highlighters are denser than luminizing lotions, so use them only on areas you want to highlight, like the inner corners of YOUR EYES, the cupid's bow of THE LIPS, and under YOUR BROW BONES.

89

Slim your nose by using cream shimmer to draw a line down its length; the product reflects light, creating the illusion of STRAIGHTER BONE STRUCTURE.

90

RED-CARPET SECRET

"EVERY WOMAN— EVEN WOMEN OF COLOR— SHOULD WEAR A BLUSH BRONZER. NOT A SELF-TANNER, A BRONZER!" —IMAN

Q&A

BURNING QUESTIONS, FINALLY ANSWERED

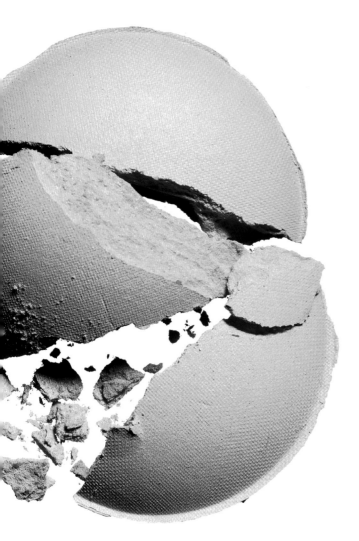

HOW CAN I TONE DOWN TOO MUCH BLUSH?

If you've overdone it with too much cream blush, blot the color off with a tissue. If powder blush is the cause of the problem, diffuse it with translucent powder; dust it on with a brush or powder puff and smooth it across your cheeks until the color is subdued. Since gel and liquid blush "stain" the cheeks, the only way to lighten them is to wash your face, moisturize, and reapply your makeup more sparingly.

I HAVE VERY DARK SKIN, AND BLUSH NEVER SEEMS TO SHOW UP ON ME. DO YOU HAVE ANY TIPS?

The darker your skin, the brighter the blush should be—that way, it reads on your face. Try a bright red or cranberry blush, says makeup artist Billy B., who has worked with Rosario Dawson and Tyra Banks. On very dark women, like model Alek Wek, they are appropriate and flattering. In addition, because the products are deeply pigmented, there's no risk that the color will look ashy on deep complexions. Don't feel, however, that you must wear blush just for the sake of wearing it. Women with darker skin often look great with just bronzer.

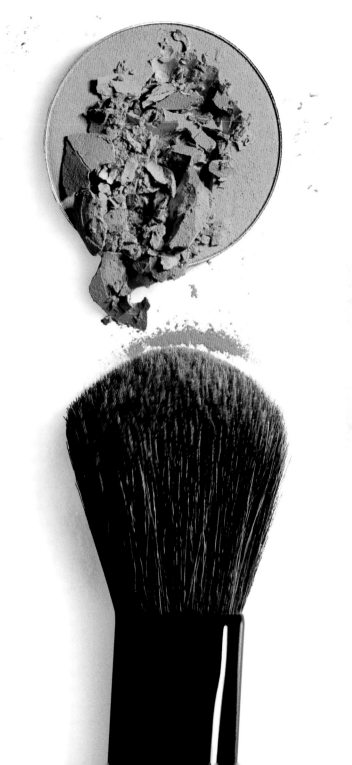

MY FACE HAS A LOT OF REDNESS. CAN I STILL WEAR BLUSH?

Absolutely, says makeup artist Sue Devitt, who has worked with Diane Lane, Eva Longoria Parker, and Brooke Shields. As a preliminary step, neutralize the redness with a yellow-based tinted moisturizer or foundation before adding cheek color. After applying the base, use a pink or slightly brownish blush over foundation; this will give a healthy flush without imparting more red tones to your skin.

A MAKEUP ARTIST SUGGESTED I TRY A NEON-PINK BLUSH. CAN I PULL THIS OFF IN REAL LIFE?

"Fear not," says N.Y.C. makeup artist Gita Bass, who has worked with Tina Fey, Debra Messing, and Elizabeth Banks. "When it's used correctly, the result can be quite beautiful and natural-looking." The key is to pick the right formula for your complexion. While medium and dark skin tones can handle a pigment-packed cream blush, lighter ones should opt for a powder formula, which goes on sheer and is easy to blend. To apply, focus the color on the apples of the cheeks and swipe upward. And keep the rest of the face neutral to avoid looking overly made-up.

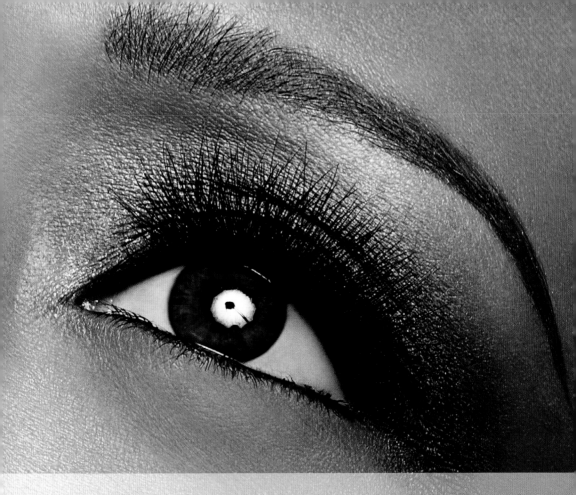

Eyes

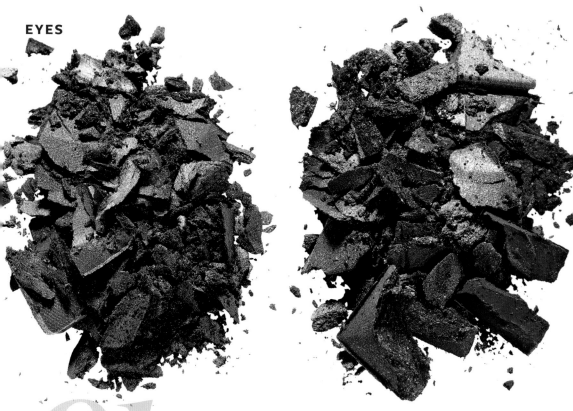

91

To make eyes really stand out,

wear an eye shadow that's the opposite of your eye shade on the color spectrum: PEACHY BROWN HUES bring out blue eyes. Blue tints flatter both dark and light brown eyes; the darker your eyes, the darker the blue you should choose. EARTHY TONES, like reddish browns, complement green eyes best. Lavender and plum pigments amp up hazel eyes.

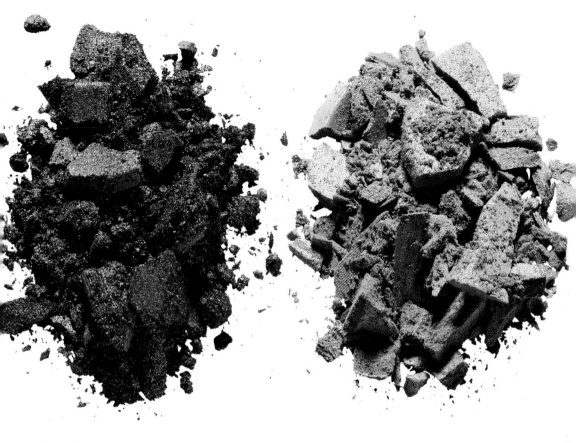

92

Choose eye shadow powders that feel smooth, not dusty to the touch, since powders can sometimes look cakey and exaggerate lines. Apply with a SOFT, DOMED SHADOW BRUSH to blend into creases and corners.

93

To highlight lids, choose a light-reflecting metallic or SHIMMERY EYE SHADOW. Or, to create depth, look for one that is matte.

94

"FOR A SMOKY EYE, MOISTURIZE THE AREA FIRST, SO WHEN YOU LINE THE LID WITH A PENCIL IT WILL SMUDGE NATURALLY."
—ELLEN POMPEO

95

For rich pigmentation and long-lasting coverage, wet a shadow brush and use it to apply powder shadow over your lids; the WET BRUSH INTENSIFIES THE COLOR and will help the powder stick.

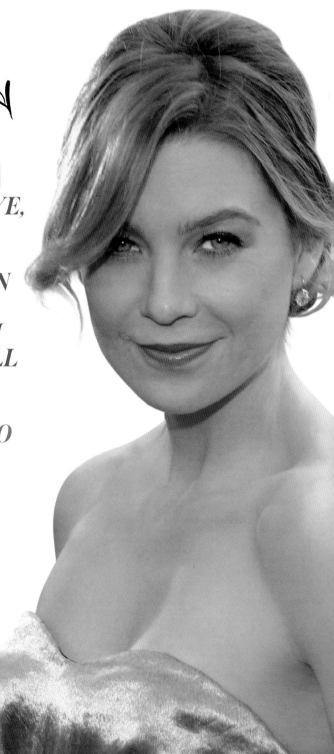

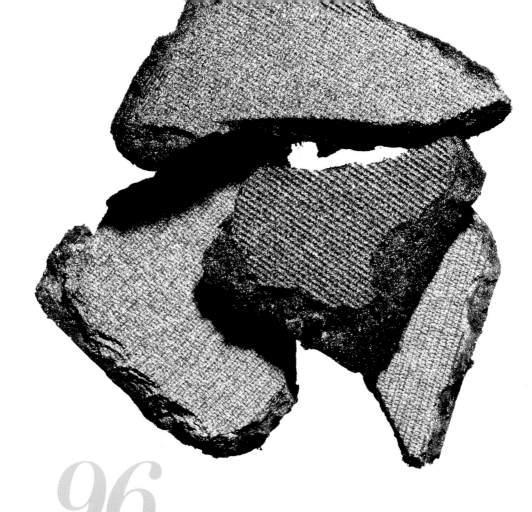

96

A truly dramatic eye requires more than two shades.

"You need three for depth," says makeup artist Chantel Miller, who likes a CHARCOAL SHADOW ON LIDS, a darker gunmetal along lash lines, and a silvery gray blended from the crease to BELOW THE BROWS.

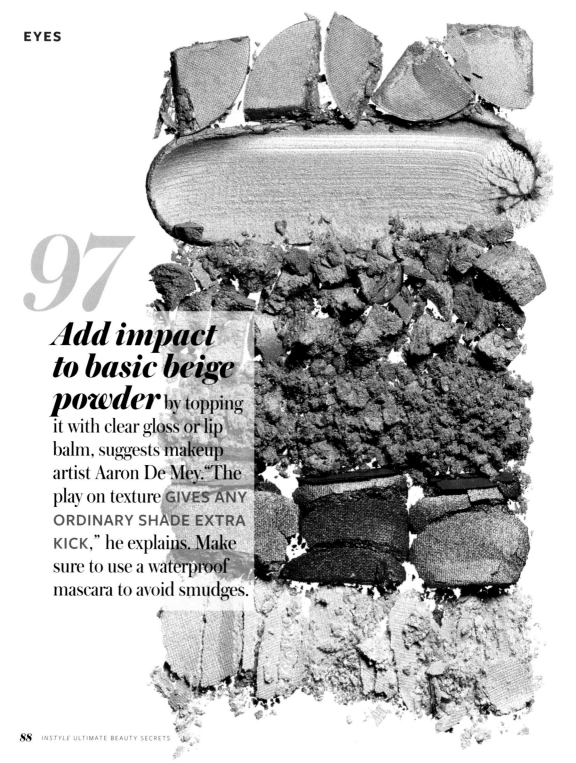

97

Add impact to basic beige powder by topping it with clear gloss or lip balm, suggests makeup artist Aaron De Mey. "The play on texture GIVES ANY ORDINARY SHADE EXTRA KICK," he explains. Make sure to use a waterproof mascara to avoid smudges.

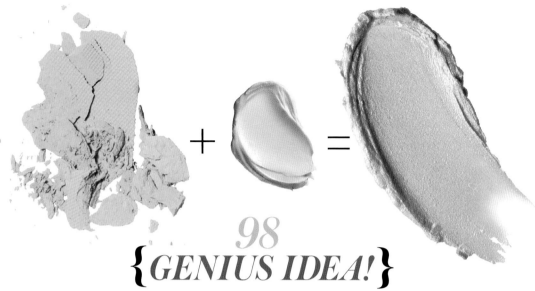

{*GENIUS IDEA!*}

Fix messy, cracked eye shadow by popping it out of its tray, putting it into a makeup palette, and crushing it. Add a dab of Vaseline or eye cream until you've gotten the right consistency. Voilà! Cream shadow.

99

For a subtle look, choose a cream shadow, which melts onto skin. Just be careful if you have oily skin: CREAMS CAN SLIDE around and gather in creases.

100

Sparkly gold shadow is a chic alternative to classic browns and beiges. "It's a subtle way to upgrade your look," says Blake Lively's makeup artist Amy Tagliamonti. "But you don't want to look OVERLY MADE-UP, so keep the rest of your face shimmer-free."

101

For a creamy eye shadow that won't crease, use a waterproof eyeliner pencil instead of shadow. Draw it OVER YOUR EYELID, then blend with YOUR FINGER.

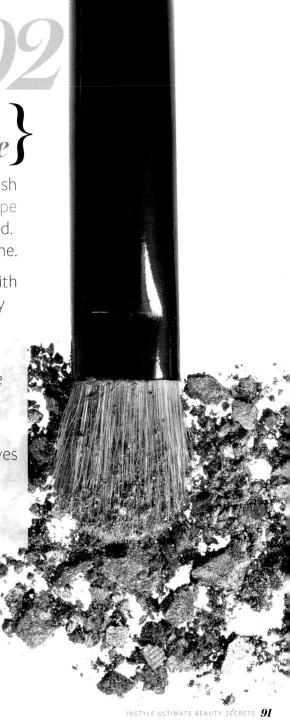

102

{ **the perfect ...**
classic smoky eye }

1. Use a medium-size round brush to apply powder in an arch shape just above the crease of the lid. Then blend down to the lash line.

2. Trace the upper lash line with a soft black pencil, then gently smudge with your fingertip.

3. With a smaller, firm-bristle brush, press a gunmetal shade into the lower lash line.

4. Apply a pale silver powder to the inner corners of the eyes to lighten the overall effect.

5. Pile on mascara.

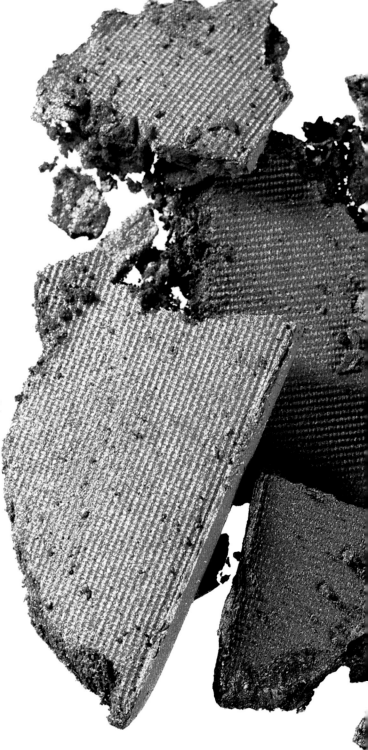

103

Purple is a modern take on the smoky eye.

Apply pale violet shadow on lids, then blend a dark plum shadow into the creases. Rim LOWER LASHES WITH BLACK LINER and top with a layer of lilac shadow applied with a wet brush.

104

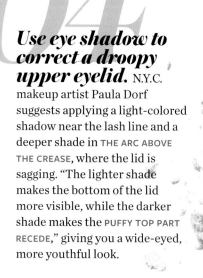

Use eye shadow to correct a droopy upper eyelid. N.Y.C. makeup artist Paula Dorf suggests applying a light-colored shadow near the lash line and a deeper shade in THE ARC ABOVE THE CREASE, where the lid is sagging. "The lighter shade makes the bottom of the lid more visible, while the darker shade makes the PUFFY TOP PART RECEDE," giving you a wide-eyed, more youthful look.

105

Erase shadow mistakes without ruining your makeup: Dip a cotton swab in concealer, then SKIM IT OVER THE SKIN. The concealer will pick up shadow without smudging.

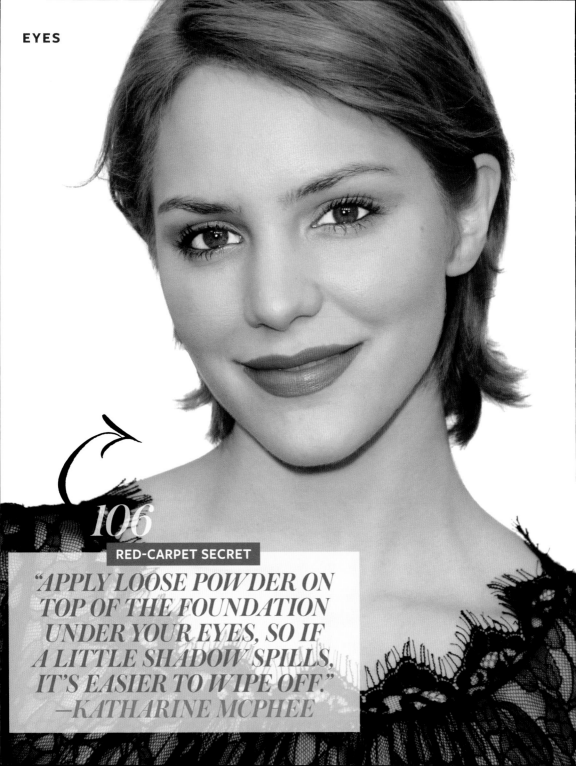

106

RED-CARPET SECRET

"APPLY LOOSE POWDER ON TOP OF THE FOUNDATION UNDER YOUR EYES, SO IF A LITTLE SHADOW SPILLS, IT'S EASIER TO WIPE OFF."
—KATHARINE MCPHEE

107

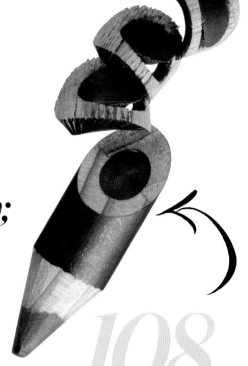

Apply liner after shadow; shadow can dull the liner, so it's best to DO IT SECOND for the most impact.

108

Always sharpen a pencil to REMOVE ANY BACTERIA before lining eyes.

109

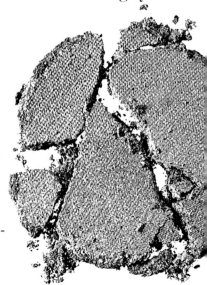

For the most natural-looking liner, use powder liner, which is DENSELY PIGMENTED, and apply with a liner brush or ANY FINE, SHORT-BRISTLE BRUSH.

110

Kohl pencil liners are highly versatile:

Because they are fatter and softer than more-precise liquid or SHARP-TIPPED LINER PENCILS, they work well for a smoky eye. Or you can USE THEM ALONE for a soft daytime look.

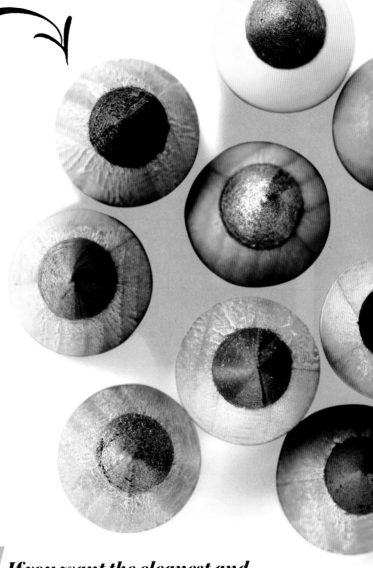

111

If you want the cleanest and longest-lasting liner, opt for liquid eyeliner. It's a defined look that requires a steady hand. To apply it, start at the MIDDLE OF YOUR UPPER LASH LINE and move outward, then draw from the inner corner BACK TO THE MIDDLE.

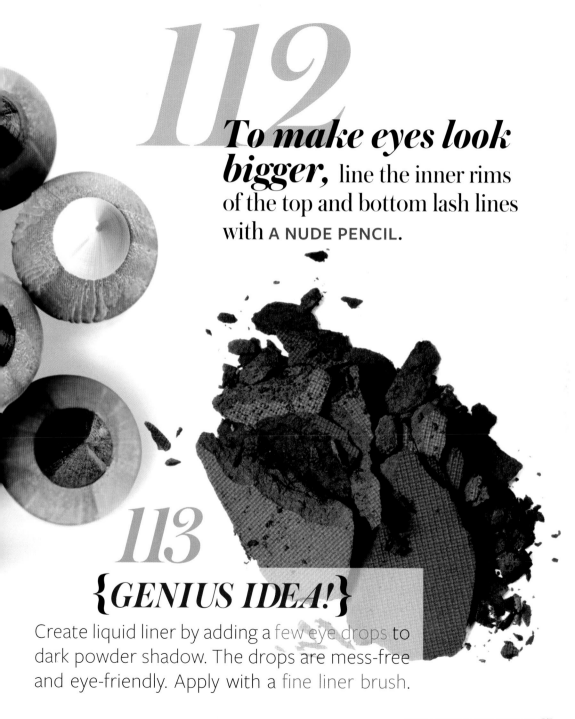

112

To make eyes look bigger, line the inner rims of the top and bottom lash lines with A NUDE PENCIL.

113

{GENIUS IDEA!}

Create liquid liner by adding a few eye drops to dark powder shadow. The drops are mess-free and eye-friendly. Apply with a fine liner brush.

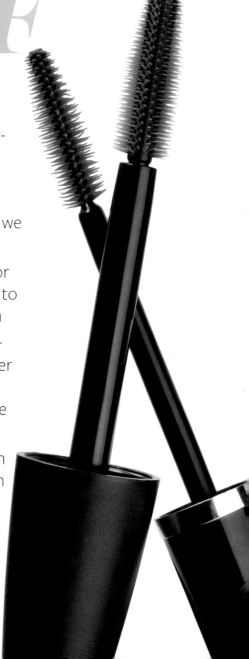

114

{ *4 ways to*
perk up eyes }

1. DARK CIRCLES Consider taking a low-dose antihistamine (check with your doctor first). "Allergens are a major trigger for undereye shadows," says dermatologist Tina Alster. "As we age we become more reactive to them."

2. PUFFINESS Place a cold compress or cold cucumber slices on eyes for five to 10 minutes, then pat on an eye cream or gel that's been stored in the fridge.

3. TIRED EYES Use your pinkie or a liner brush to dab a light cream shadow at the inner corner of each eye, then line inner rims with a nude pencil.

4. REDNESS Apply black mascara, then tip the ends of your lashes with plum or navy mascara to make the whites of the eyes look brighter. Or just smudge a bit of deep navy eyeliner on the inner rims of the upper lids.

115

When the temperatures rise, consider using *cream blush* as an eye shadow, says makeup artist Francesca Tolot. The warmest season is all about bright colors, so a coral, rose or pink shade looks fresh on eyes. The key, though, is to *keep it light*—one coat blended with your fingers should do it—as sweat can lead to creasing.

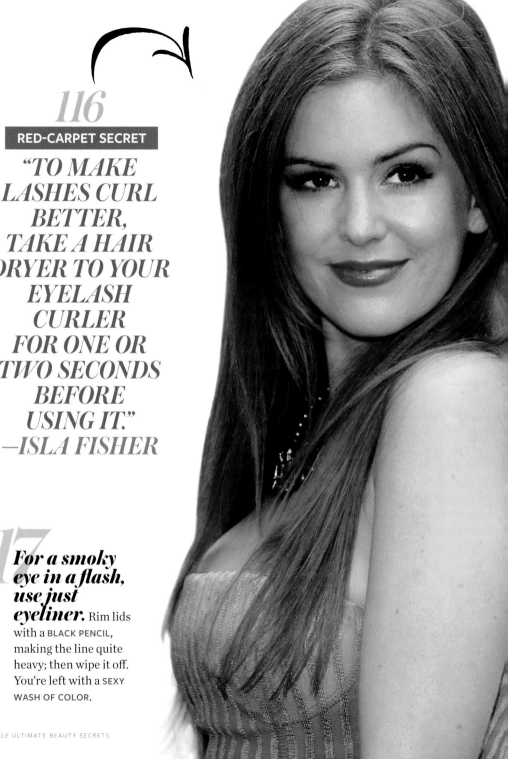

116

"TO MAKE LASHES CURL BETTER, TAKE A HAIR DRYER TO YOUR EYELASH CURLER FOR ONE OR TWO SECONDS BEFORE USING IT."
—ISLA FISHER

117 **For a smoky eye in a flash, use just eyeliner.** Rim lids with a BLACK PENCIL, making the line quite heavy; then wipe it off. You're left with a SEXY WASH OF COLOR.

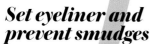

Set eyeliner and prevent smudges by using a tiny brush to dust TRANSLUCENT POWDER over liner.

118

119

Before applying mascara, curl lashes. "Curling your lashes is the easiest thing you can do to make your EYES LOOK BIGGER," says makeup artist Troy Surratt, who has worked on Fergie and Hilary Duff. To create a soft, lasting curve, squeeze the curler THREE TIMES, moving from roots to tips.

120

Never pump your mascara.
Forcing the wand into the tube and pulling it out quickly pushes air into it, DRYING OUT THE MASCARA.

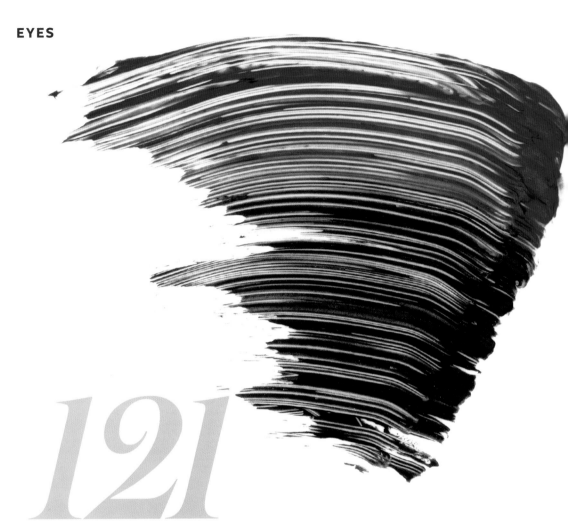

121

To create thickness, hold your mascara wand horizontally at the base of the lashes and wiggle it back and forth FROM UNDERNEATH before drawing it up and out to the tips. You can also USE A THICKENING FORMULA, which has waxes that coat the lashes, bulking them up.

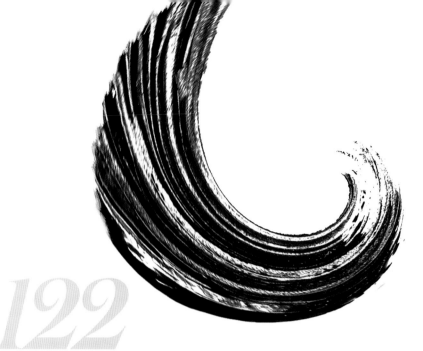

122

Curling mascara formulas

are good for shorter lashes, which can be HARD TO GRAB WITH A LASH CURLER. The mascara contracts, causing lashes to SHRINK AND LIFT.

123

Get the most mascara onto your lashes with

every swipe by using a lengthening formula. Its wand comes with DENSELY PACKED BRISTLES for getting pigment onto every lash. The design also makes it easier to touch up the tips, the most important area to coat for THE APPEARANCE OF LONG LASHES.

To avoid smudges when applying mascara, hold a

spoon (plastic works well, and you won't miss it from the kitchen) above the UPPER LASHES and then under the lower lashes to shield the REST OF YOUR MAKEUP.

124

125

During the day, skip mascara on

the lower lashes entirely—"it can look TOO DRAMATIC," says makeup artist Molly R. Stern, who has worked with Leighton Meester and Mandy Moore. Instead, dot A DARK BROWN PENCIL between lashes to make them look fuller.

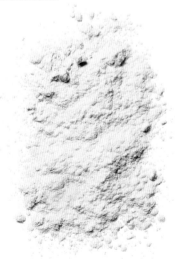

126

For extra-thick eyelashes, dust lashes first

with TRANSLUCENT POWDER, then apply mascara.

127

Elongate eyes by using dark brown mascara on the

INNER HALF OF THE EYE and black mascara on the outer lashes.

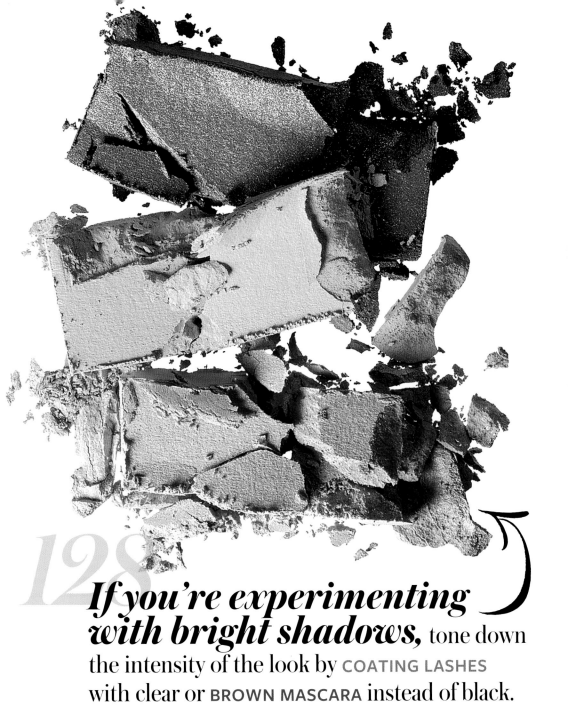

128 ***If you're experimenting with bright shadows,*** tone down the intensity of the look by COATING LASHES with clear or BROWN MASCARA instead of black.

129
{ Special Occasion Secret }

Fake lashes really make eyes pop. Curl your natural lashes and apply all eye makeup but mascara. Keep in mind that your false lashes should complement the level of intensity of the rest of your makeup.

FOR A NATURAL LOOK Use individual clusters. Pick up each cluster with tweezers, dip the end into glue, wait 20 seconds for the glue to get tacky, and apply from the center of the eye to the outside corner; four clusters per eye is plenty.

FOR A DRAMATIC LOOK Use a medium-length strip. Pick up the strip with tweezers, dip it in glue, wait 20 seconds, then lay the strip on your lash line and pinch together with fingertips.

FOR AN EXTREME LOOK Use a full strip. Roll the lashes between your fingertips to loosen the bend and make them more comfortable to wear. Use a toothpick to apply glue to the strip, wait 20 seconds, then apply the strip starting at the outer corner. After applying, use black liquid liner to emphasize the lash line.

Whatever style you choose, finish the look by waiting for the false lashes to dry, then applying mascara.

130

To thoroughly remove mascara, wrap a cotton pad in a tissue and saturate with oil-based remover. The tissue prevents the cotton from LEAVING LINT BEHIND. Hold the pad over your eye for five seconds, then swipe up, down, and toward the outer corner of the eye. Finally, wash your face with your REGULAR FACIAL CLEANSER.

131

If you tweeze your own brows, keep your face shape in mind. MOST FACES LOOK BEST WITH A CLASSIC BROW SHAPE: medium full with a tapered end and soft arch. Round faces benefit from stronger brows with a high arch to add angles to the face. Heart-shaped faces look great with a less noticeable arch and a natural, full look. Long faces are flattered by straighter brows, which add the illusion of fullness. Square faces should use a low arch to soften angles.

132

Tweeze brows after showering.

Hot steam opens the pores so plucking is less painful. Or if you are in a rush, PRESS A WARM WASHCLOTH to the area to relax the follicles, and grab each hair CLOSE TO THE ROOT, softly pulling one at a time.

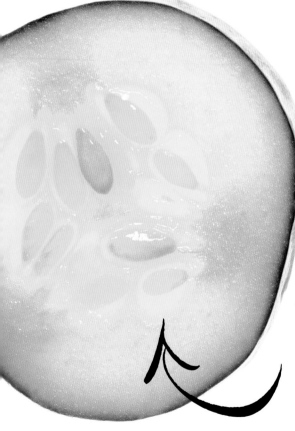

133

If you are super sensitive, numb the area first by pressing A BAG OF FROZEN PEAS against your brow for about TWO MINUTES BEFORE PLUCKING.

134

After tweezing, swipe brows with rubbing alcohol to prevent ingrown hairs, then REDUCE REDNESS by applying COLD CUCUMBER SLICES or chilled green-tea bags.

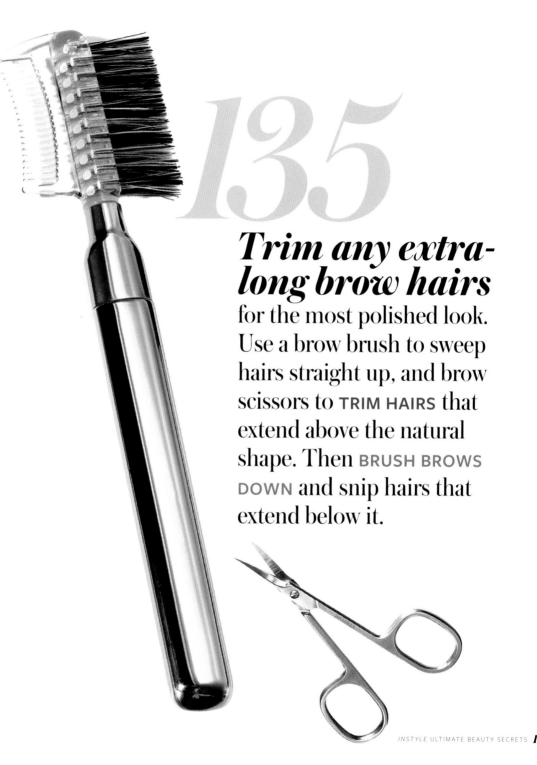

135

Trim any extra-long brow hairs

for the most polished look. Use a brow brush to sweep hairs straight up, and brow scissors to TRIM HAIRS that extend above the natural shape. Then BRUSH BROWS DOWN and snip hairs that extend below it.

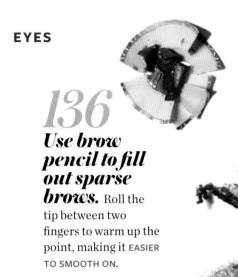

136

Use brow pencil to fill out sparse brows. Roll the tip between two fingers to warm up the point, making it EASIER TO SMOOTH ON.

137

Use brow powder
instead of a pencil to extend A SHORT EYEBROW. Pencil can look waxy and fake when not obscured by brow hairs. Set color with CLEAR BROW GEL.

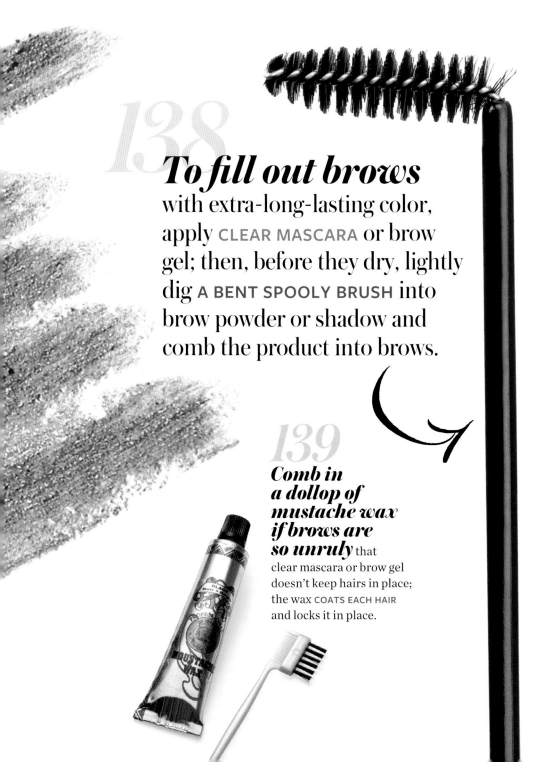

138

To fill out brows

with extra-long-lasting color, apply CLEAR MASCARA or brow gel; then, before they dry, lightly dig A BENT SPOOLY BRUSH into brow powder or shadow and comb the product into brows.

139

Comb in a dollop of mustache wax if brows are so unruly that clear mascara or brow gel doesn't keep hairs in place; the wax COATS EACH HAIR and locks it in place.

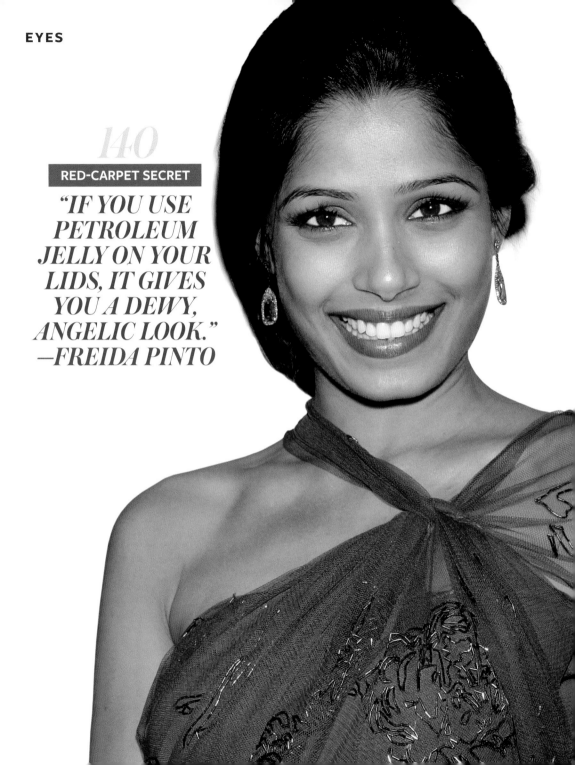

140

RED-CARPET SECRET

"IF YOU USE PETROLEUM JELLY ON YOUR LIDS, IT GIVES YOU A DEWY, ANGELIC LOOK."
—FREIDA PINTO

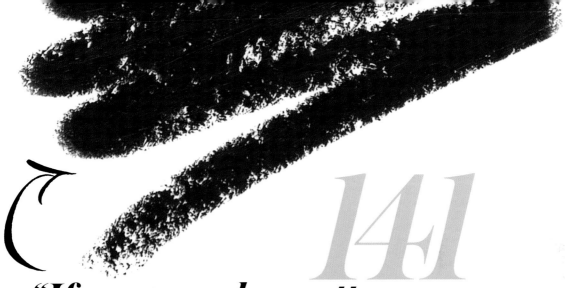

141

"If you are a brunette, your brows should be two shades lighter than your hair," says brow guru DAMONE ROBERTS, who has worked with Megan Fox. "If you have blond or red hair, they should be ONE SHADE DARKER."

142

To lighten brows, use an at-home color kit that's lighter than your hair; you'll get a more natural-looking result than with at-home bleaching. DAB AQUAPHOR AROUND BROWS first to protect skin.

143

To darken light brows, brush them up and out with a clean spooly, then use a pointed TAUPE BROW PENCIL (for fair brows) or a brown one (for darker brows) to draw tiny, feathery strokes on the skin beneath the hairs. Finally, GO OVER BROWS WITH AN ANGLE-CUT BRUSH, blending and smoothing out the color across the area.

Q&A

BURNING QUESTIONS, FINALLY ANSWERED

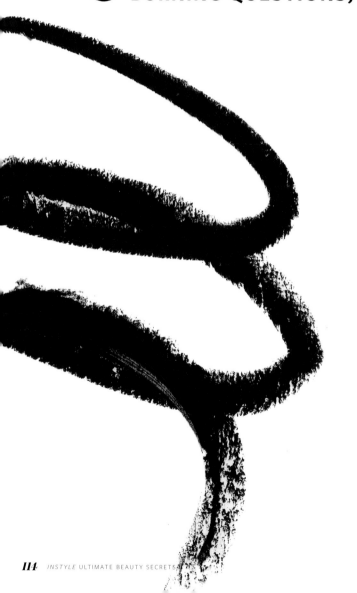

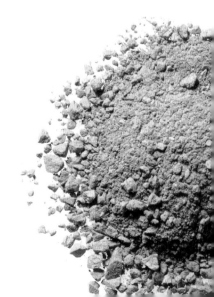

MY HANDS ALWAYS SHAKE WHEN I APPLY EYELINER, WHICH LEADS TO CROOKED LINES. WHAT CAN I DO TO STAY STEADY?
For stability, rest your elbow on a table in front of a mirror, and with your free hand, pull your lid taut at the outside corner of the eye to create a smooth, flat canvas. For added security, lay a mirror flat on a table in front of you so you are forced to look down. You'll have a clearer view of your entire lid and be able to get the makeup closer to (or right into) the lash line. Clean up a crooked line with a moistened cotton swab.

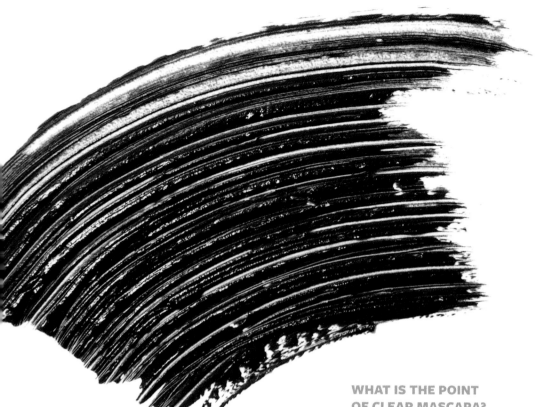

MY EYE MAKEUP ALWAYS RUNS. HOW CAN I PREVENT THIS?

Before applying any kind of liner, prep your upper and lower lids with a minuscule amount of foundation and set it with translucent powder. This creates a dry, grease-free surface. After you've applied liner, another dusting of translucent powder will hold it in place. If you prefer not to layer on the foundation and powder, set liner by tracing powder shadow (in the same shade) directly on top of it. For super-long-lasting liner, try this: Stroke on a pencil liner first, apply powder liner (or shadow) over that, and top it all off with liquid liner.

WHAT IS THE POINT OF CLEAR MASCARA?

Clear mascara is like lip gloss for your lashes. It makes them look darker and more visible without being obvious. It's also great for people with oily skin, since it won't smudge. Clear mascara can also be used as brow gel to hold unruly brows in place.

WHAT KIND OF MASCARA WON'T IRRITATE SENSITIVE EYES?

Large particles (like hard waxes and fibers), fragrances, and harsh preservatives are the major eye irritants. Always read the label before you buy, and opt for mascaras that are 100 percent fragrance-free and dermatologist-, ophthalmologist-, and/or allergy-tested.

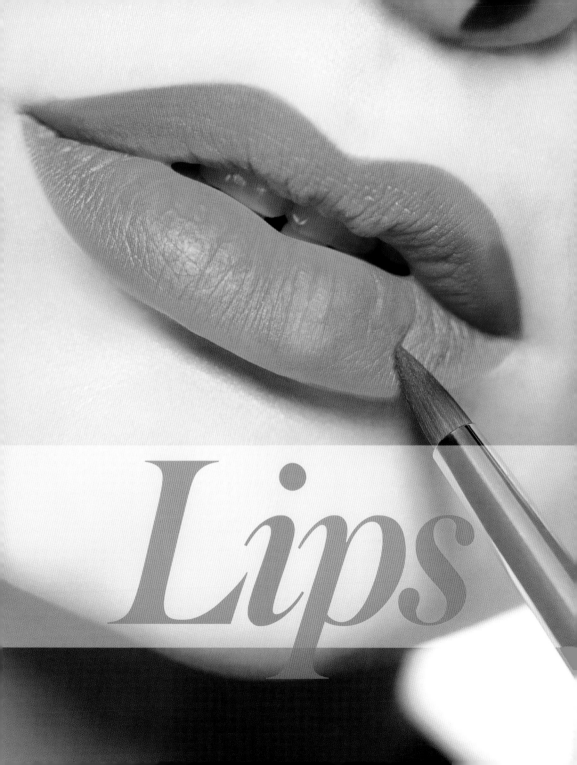

Lips

144

Apply a balm immediately after getting out of the shower, when your lips are STILL A LITTLE MOIST; this will create a smooth surface once you're READY FOR COLOR.

145

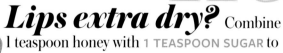

Lips extra dry? Combine 1 teaspoon honey with 1 TEASPOON SUGAR to exfoliate them, says makeup artist Kristofer Buckle, who helped polish looks for Christina Aguilera and Jennifer Connelly. He blends the two ingredients in his hand, then applies the mixture in A CIRCULAR MOTION for 90 seconds before wiping it off.

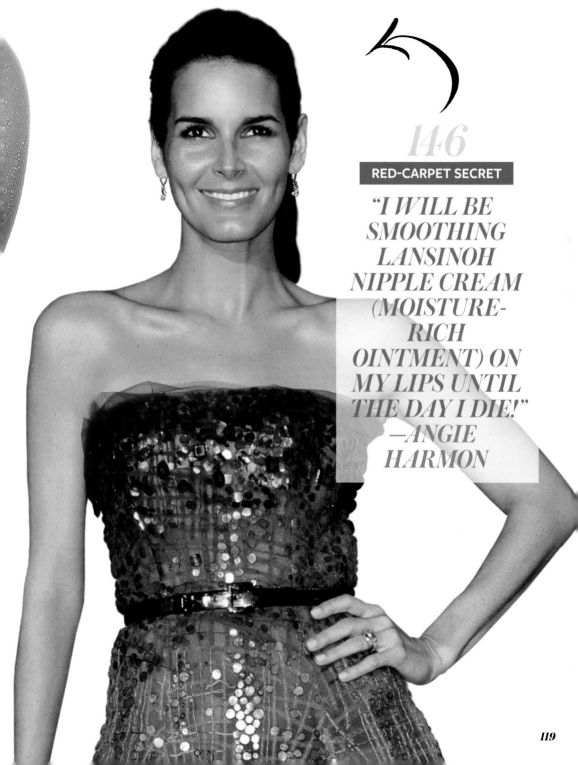

RED-CARPET SECRET

"I WILL BE SMOOTHING LANSINOH NIPPLE CREAM (MOISTURE-RICH OINTMENT) ON MY LIPS UNTIL THE DAY I DIE!" —ANGIE HARMON

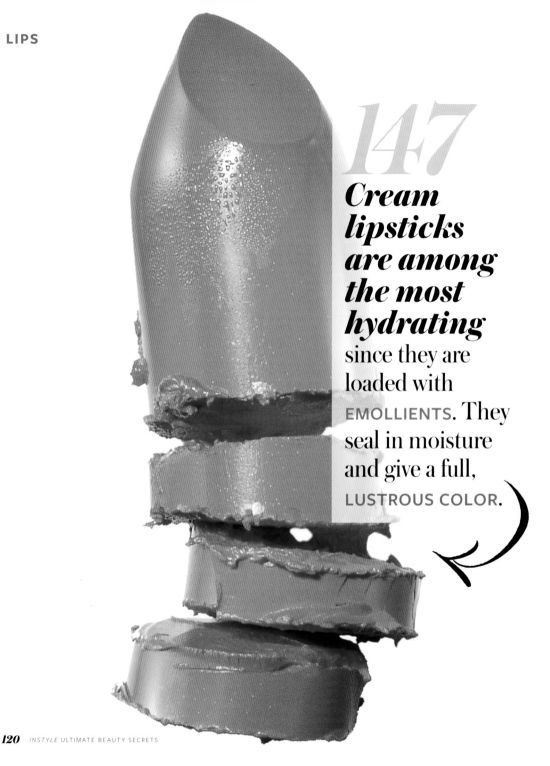

147

Cream lipsticks are among the most hydrating since they are loaded with EMOLLIENTS. They seal in moisture and give a full, LUSTROUS COLOR.

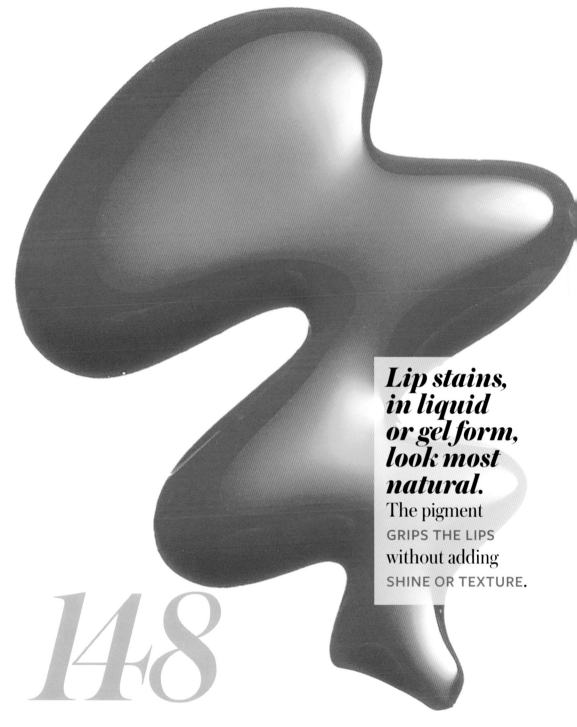

148

Lip stains, in liquid or gel form, look most natural. The pigment GRIPS THE LIPS without adding SHINE OR TEXTURE.

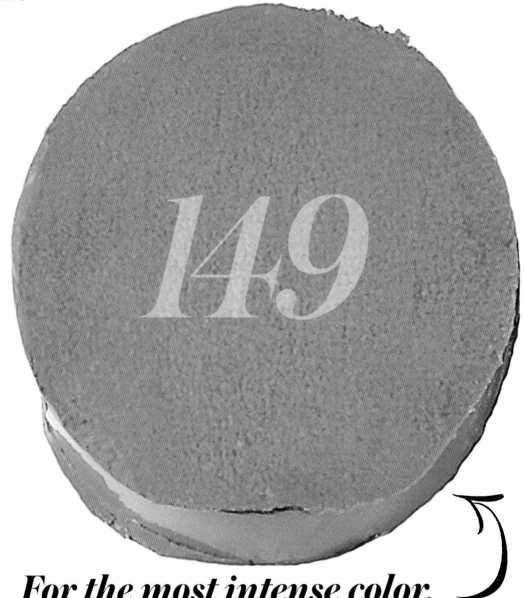

149

For the most intense color,

MATTE LIPSTICKS are the way to go. They are SATURATED WITH PIGMENT and have no shine.

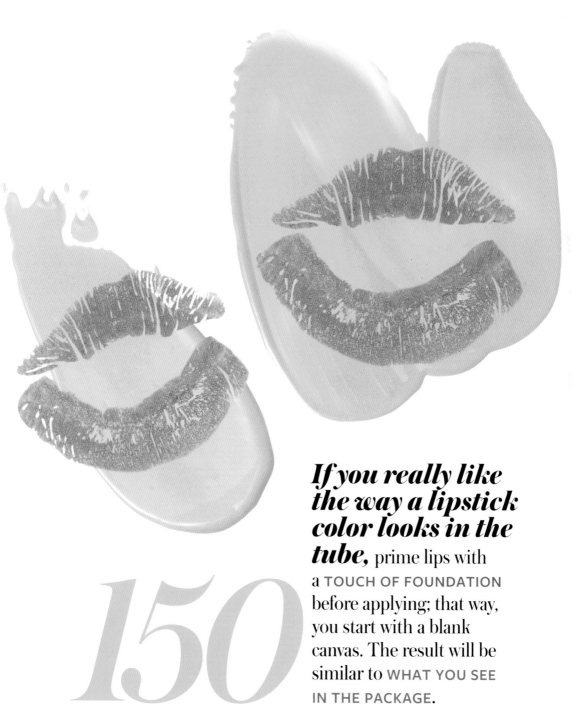

If you really like the way a lipstick color looks in the tube, prime lips with a TOUCH OF FOUNDATION before applying; that way, you start with a blank canvas. The result will be similar to WHAT YOU SEE IN THE PACKAGE.

150

151

The best nude, pink and red for fair, medium and dark complexions:

FAIR SKIN looks best in pinky nudes, subtle pale pinks, and cherry reds. MEDIUM COMPLEXIONS are flattered by yellow- or orange-based nudes, vibrant pinks, and classic tomato reds. DARKER SKIN TONES also benefit from yellow- or orange-based nudes, as well as bold berries and fuchsias, and earthy, brick reds.

152

Yes, redheads can wear red lips!

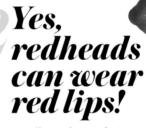

Redheads with ivory skin should stick to bluish red lip color. Those with peachy complexions and strawberry-blond hair look great in red lipsticks that are golden based.

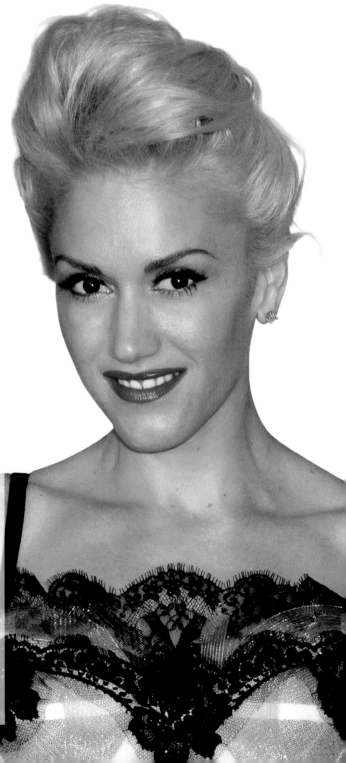

153

"I LOVE TO LAYER TONS OF DIFFERENT SHADES TO CREATE NEW COLORS. I START WITH MATTE LIPSTICK THAT'S REALLY DRY, THEN I PUT A MORE CREAMY, MOIST LIPSTICK ON TOP. AND MY TRICK FOR NOT GETTING IT ON MY TEETH? BE REALLY CAREFUL!"
—GWEN STEFANI

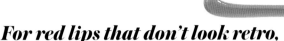

154

For red lips that don't look retro, FILL IN LIPS with red pencil, add a clear balm, and blot for A NATURAL FINISH.

155

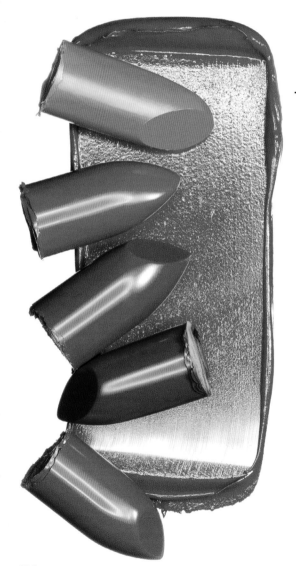

{ *the perfect ...* *classic red lips* }

1. Fill in lips with a liner that matches your lip color.

2. Apply red color straight from the tube just to the center of lips.

3. Using a lip brush, blend color evenly out to the corners.

4. Blot, then repeat steps 2 and 3 for an extra-long-lasting finish.

5. To make sure no color gets on your teeth, wash your index finger, place your lips in a small o shape, insert your finger, and pull it out. Any lipstick that is on the opening of your lips will come off on your finger, not your teeth.

156

If your skin has ruddy undertones or gets *extra blotchy* and flushed in the heat, consider *skipping bold red* lip colors. The red lip pigment will end up emphasizing your skin's redness. Stick to *soft pinks* and nudes instead.

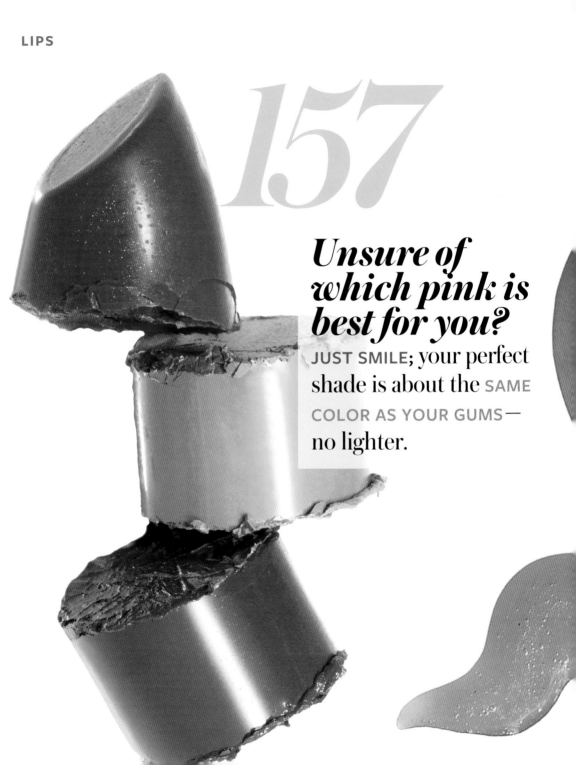

157

Unsure of which pink is best for you?

JUST SMILE; your perfect shade is about the SAME COLOR AS YOUR GUMS— no lighter.

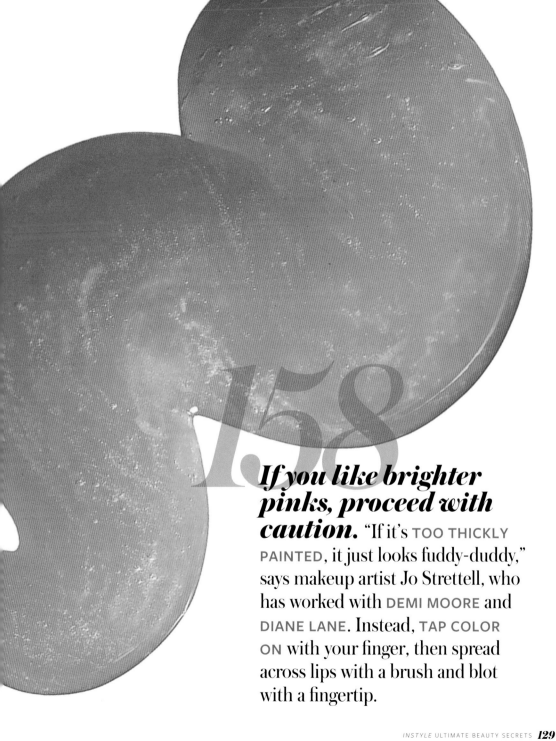

158

If you like brighter pinks, proceed with caution. "If it's TOO THICKLY PAINTED, it just looks fuddy-duddy," says makeup artist Jo Strettell, who has worked with DEMI MOORE and DIANE LANE. Instead, TAP COLOR ON with your finger, then spread across lips with a brush and blot with a fingertip.

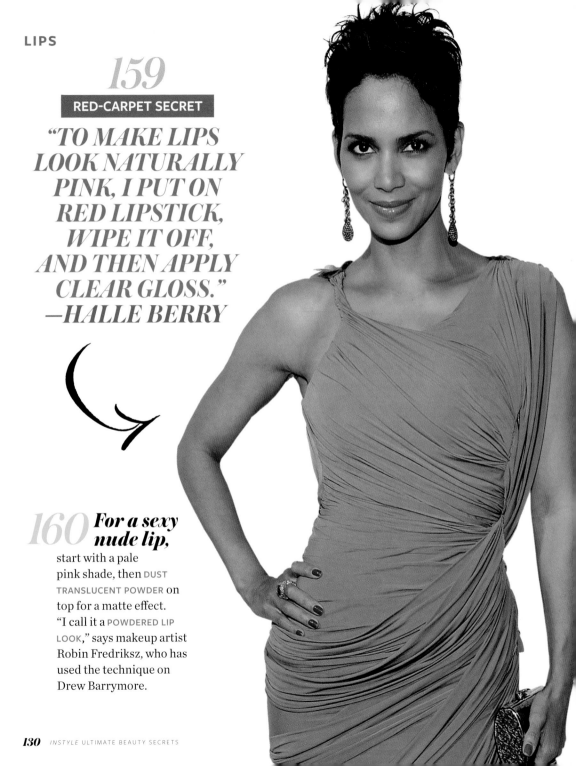

159

RED-CARPET SECRET

"TO MAKE LIPS LOOK NATURALLY PINK, I PUT ON RED LIPSTICK, WIPE IT OFF, AND THEN APPLY CLEAR GLOSS."
—HALLE BERRY

160 **For a sexy nude lip,** start with a pale pink shade, then DUST TRANSLUCENT POWDER on top for a matte effect. "I call it a POWDERED LIP LOOK," says makeup artist Robin Fredriksz, who has used the technique on Drew Barrymore.

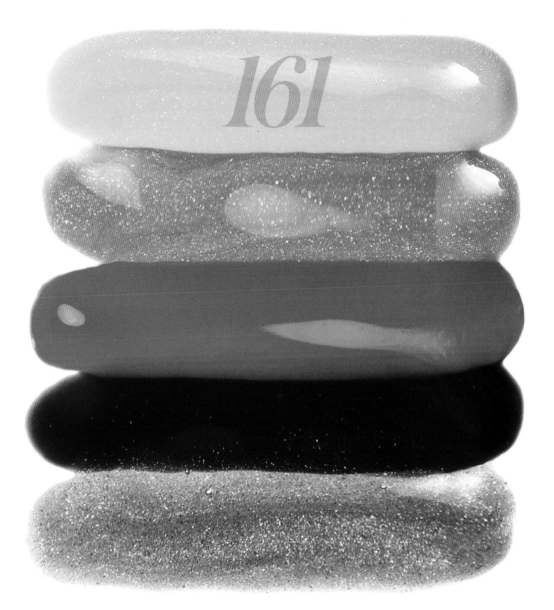

161

Turn any lip color into a shimmery new shade: Swipe sheer GOLDEN LIP GLOSS over lipstick. It instantly WARMS UP EVERY COLOR.

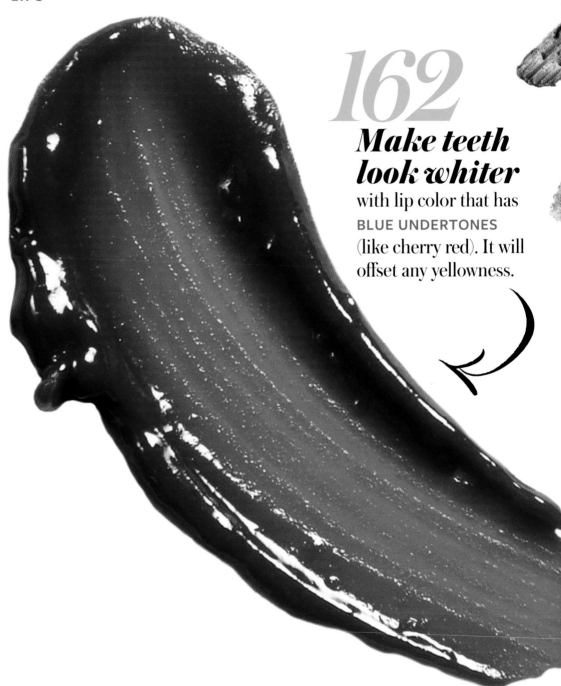

162

Make teeth look whiter

with lip color that has **BLUE UNDERTONES** (like cherry red). It will offset any yellowness.

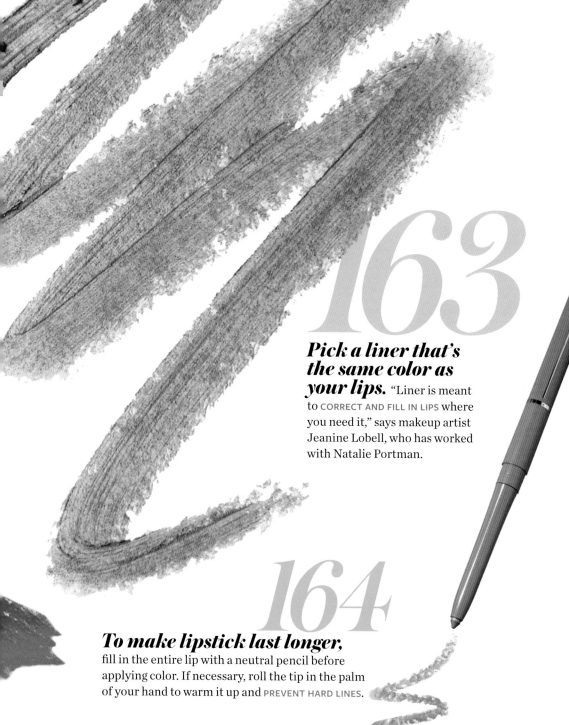

163

Pick a liner that's the same color as your lips. "Liner is meant to CORRECT AND FILL IN LIPS where you need it," says makeup artist Jeanine Lobell, who has worked with Natalie Portman.

164

To make lipstick last longer, fill in the entire lip with a neutral pencil before applying color. If necessary, roll the tip in the palm of your hand to warm it up and PREVENT HARD LINES.

165

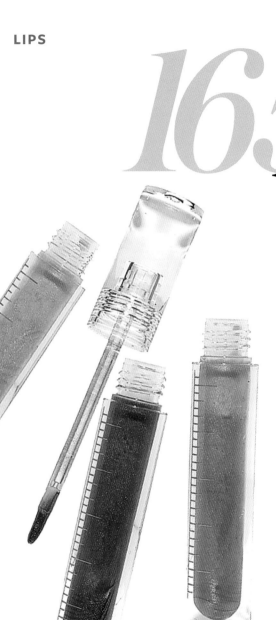

{ *3 ways to* *fake fuller lips* }

1. Dabbing peppermint oil on your lips stimulates them, causing a slight plumping effect, says Mount Kisco, N.Y., dermatologist David Bank.

2. Opt for shimmery lipsticks. They contain light-reflecting particles that make lips look fuller.

3. To add fullness to lips while wearing your favorite color, dab a bit of dusky pink or toffee-colored gloss on the center of your lower lip and your cupid's bow.

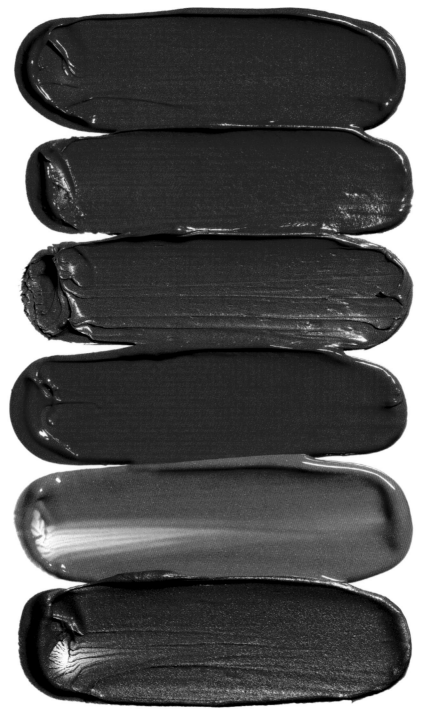

166

Give the illusion of two perfect peaks without lining lips. Just DAB CONCEALER in the groove at the center of YOUR UPPER LIP and blend well.

167

Turn any lipstick into a durable stain by blotting, reapplying, then blotting again to remove excess oils. Blot with LINT-FREE BLOTTING PAPER rather than tissue for a more natural, long-lasting look.

168

In the cold months, when lips tend to get extra dry, *keep balms accessible*. Stash one in the bathroom, your purse, your gym bag, the car, and an office drawer. N.Y.C. dermatologist Arielle Kauvar also recommends applying lip balm every time you *wash your face* and whenever you feel tempted to lick your lips. Licking them will only cause further dehydration, so resist the urge.

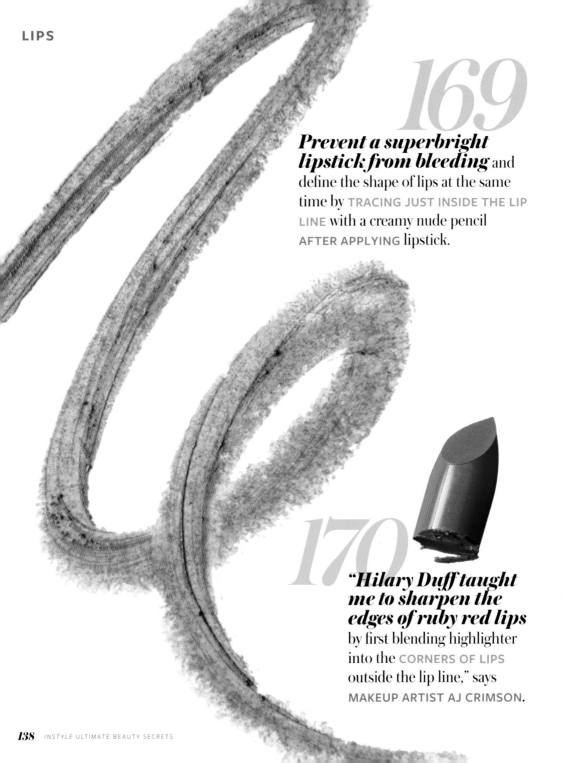

169

Prevent a superbright lipstick from bleeding and define the shape of lips at the same time by TRACING JUST INSIDE THE LIP LINE with a creamy nude pencil AFTER APPLYING lipstick.

170

"Hilary Duff taught me to sharpen the edges of ruby red lips by first blending highlighter into the CORNERS OF LIPS outside the lip line," says MAKEUP ARTIST AJ CRIMSON.

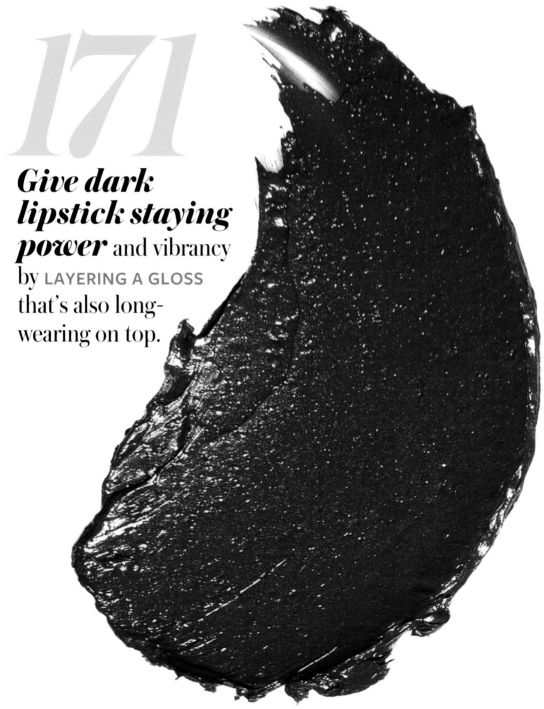

171

Give dark lipstick staying power and vibrancy by LAYERING A GLOSS that's also long-wearing on top.

Q&A

BURNING QUESTIONS, FINALLY ANSWERED

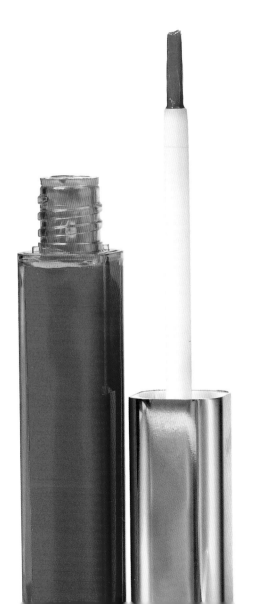

IS LIP BALM ADDICTIVE?

We've all heard the myth that certain lip treatments are spiked with addictive ingredients, which cause our lips to be incessantly chapped and in need of balm. But there's no scientific evidence to support this rumor. What seems like a physical addiction is actually a habit that happens when you get used to your lips feeling soft and supple immediately after applying balm. Without balm, your lips can seem particularly dry, so you probably start licking them to hydrate them, which in turn actually does dry them out. It's no wonder we all reach for the lip balm.

DO "TREATMENT" LIPSTICKS DO ANYTHING?

Treatment lipsticks can help to a certain extent. The amount of anti-aging product in the lipstick is minimal, so you may see a slight difference with use, but nothing significant. Typical ingredients such as vitamin C and kinetin can help prevent chapping and peeling. But the skin on the lips is extremely sensitive, so be careful: The ingredients may cause irritation. If something stings, wipe it off immediately.

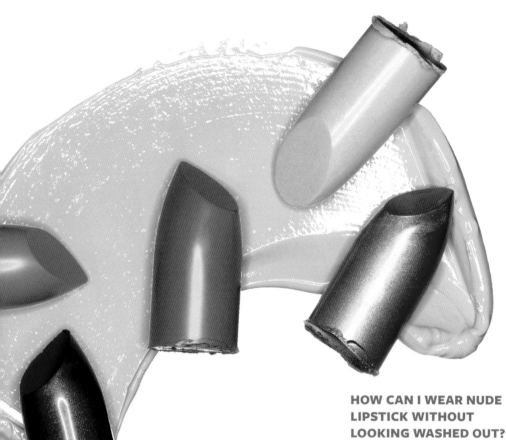

DO LIP PLUMPERS REALLY WORK?

Yes, temporarily. By stimulating the surface of the lip with ingredients such as alpha-hydroxy acids, lactic acid, or even cinnamon, many plumpers can make lips appear temporarily swollen. The effect typically lasts one to four hours. Newer plumpers contain ingredients such as hyaluronic acid, which help your lips retain moisture and therefore look plumper. But again, the effect is temporary.

HOW CAN I WEAR NUDE LIPSTICK WITHOUT LOOKING WASHED OUT?

Modern nude lips are sheer and shiny, not pasty and caked on. And actually, they're pale pink, not beige. To create a sexy nude lip, first outline your lips with a pencil one shade darker than their natural color, but avoid muddy brown hues, which are unflattering. Choose a rosy taupe if you have fair skin, a pale brick hue if you have an olive complexion, and coppery shades if you have dark skin. Then fill in lips with the pencil and top with a pale, gold-flecked sheer pink gloss. Don't glop it on: The gold flecks catch light and sparkle even if you use very little. To counteract pale lips, wear peachy or pink blush.

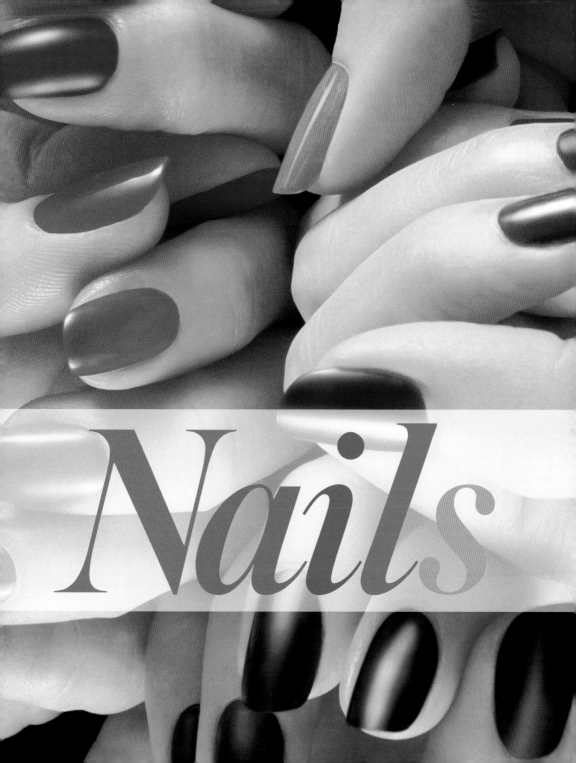

Nails

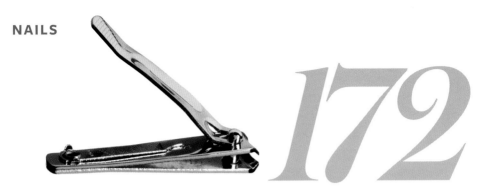

172

Trim nails with a clipper,

always STARTING AT THE SIDES. Beginning at the center can flatten THE NATURAL CURVE and cause breakage.

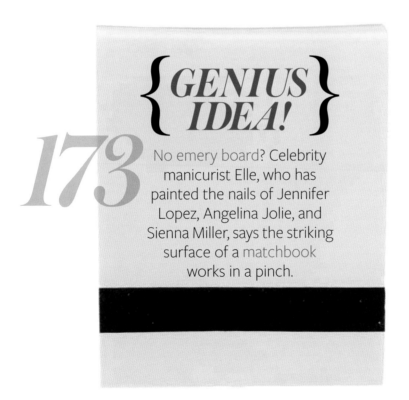

173

{ *GENIUS IDEA!* }

No emery board? Celebrity manicurist Elle, who has painted the nails of Jennifer Lopez, Angelina Jolie, and Sienna Miller, says the striking surface of a matchbook works in a pinch.

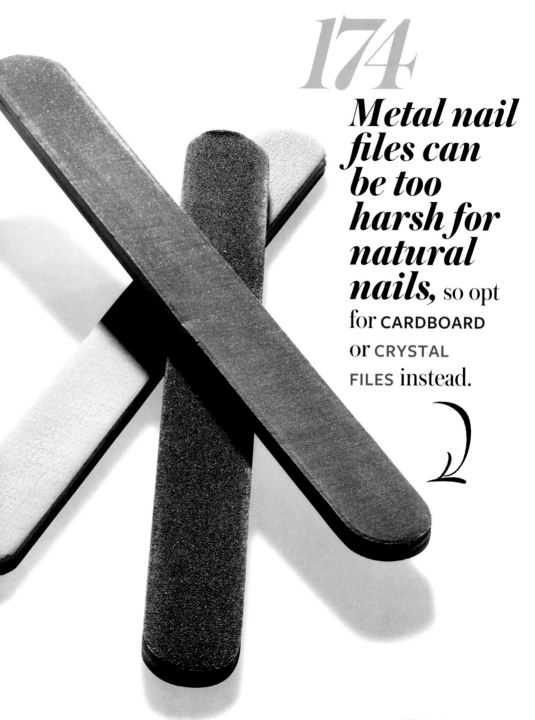

Metal nail files can be too harsh for natural nails, so opt for **CARDBOARD** or **CRYSTAL** **FILES** instead.

$\textstyle\curvearrowleft$

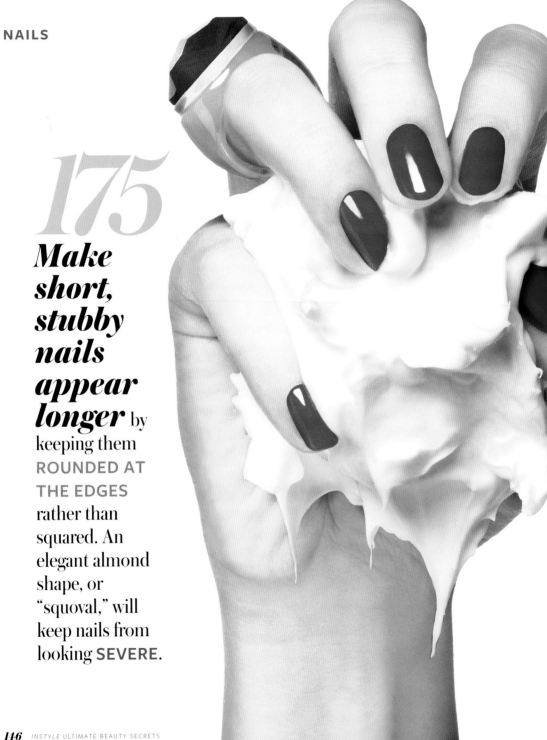

175

Make short, stubby nails appear longer by

keeping them ROUNDED AT THE EDGES rather than squared. An elegant almond shape, or "squoval," will keep nails from looking SEVERE.

176

"Toothpicks clean under the nail tip better than anything else," says L.A. makeup artist CRISTINA BARTOLUCCI, who has worked with Keri Russell. "Just be careful with the point."

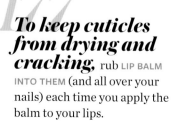

177

To keep cuticles from drying and cracking, rub LIP BALM INTO THEM (and all over your nails) each time you apply the balm to your lips.

178

To protect cuticles as you push them back,

WRAP THE TIP of your orangewood stick in a tuft of WATER-MOISTENED COTTON. The stick alone can tear cuticles.

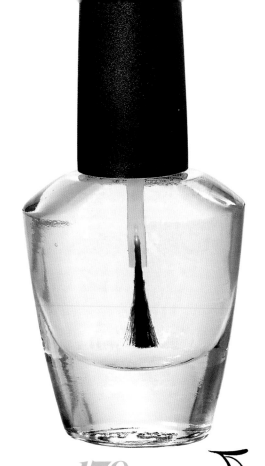

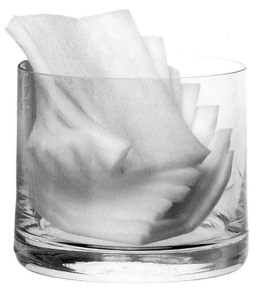

179

Use a base coat to prevent polish pigment from seeping

into nails and yellowing them. It also keeps polish from drying nails, SMOOTHS THE NAIL SURFACE, and helps polish adhere so it won't chip.

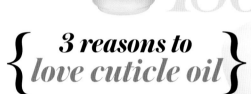

180

{ *3 reasons to*
love cuticle oil }

1. IT PROTECTS POLISH Drop
oil on each nail after polishing
to create a buffer between the
lacquer and any object that might
smudge it.

2. IT ADDS SHINE Between mani-
pedis, rub a spot of cuticle oil
onto nails; it hydrates, smooths
out imperfections, and adds a
nice sheen to lackluster nails.

**3. IT HELPS FAKE A FRENCH
MANICURE** Massage oil into nail
beds to camouflage dry skin, then
run a white nail pencil under the
rims of your nails.

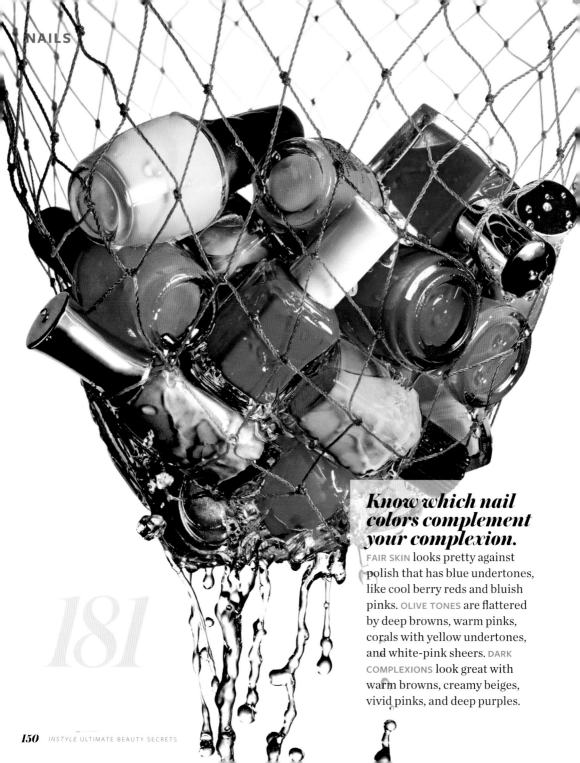

181

Know which nail colors complement your complexion.

FAIR SKIN looks pretty against polish that has blue undertones, like cool berry reds and bluish pinks. OLIVE TONES are flattered by deep browns, warm pinks, corals with yellow undertones, and white-pink sheers. DARK COMPLEXIONS look great with warm browns, creamy beiges, vivid pinks, and deep purples.

182

Give your tan a boost with an orangey nail hue, which contrasts nicely with SUN-KISSED SKIN.

183

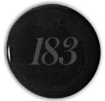

If you favor dark polish, keep nails short and groomed to avoid the CRUELLA DE VIL LOOK. Trim nails to ¼ inch past the fingertip.

184

For a finished, professional nail polish look, leave a SMALL SPACE between the CUTICLE and the POLISH LINE.

185

Rather than polishing your nail in one fell swoop, break down the process into three strokes, says N.Y.C. manicurist Bethany Newell, who has beautified Cameron Diaz's and Mary J. Blige's fingernails. First PAINT THE CENTER, then swipe along each side, KEEPING THE COATS THIN (and layering as needed) to prevent chipping.

186

Reinforce tips, since they are the first to peel. Add AN EXTRA SWIPE of base coat, color, and top coat across the EDGE OF EACH TIP.

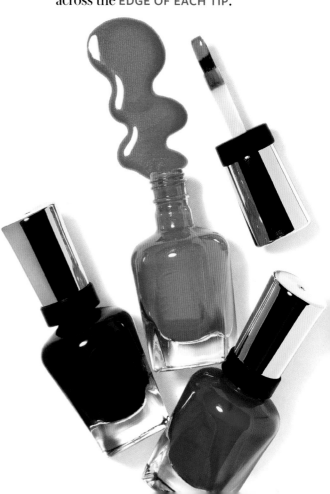

187

{ **Winter Nail Trick** }

Cool weather can make nails brittle and polish chip faster, so protect your polish by wearing gloves every time you step outside. To restore moisture to extra-dry nails, try an *at-home soak* of lemon juice, olive oil, and vitamin E oil. To maximize its absorption, remove nail polish, buff nails gently with a towel to exfoliate, then soak for five minutes. Afterward, slip on a pair of *cotton spa gloves* to keep the moisture sealed in all night.

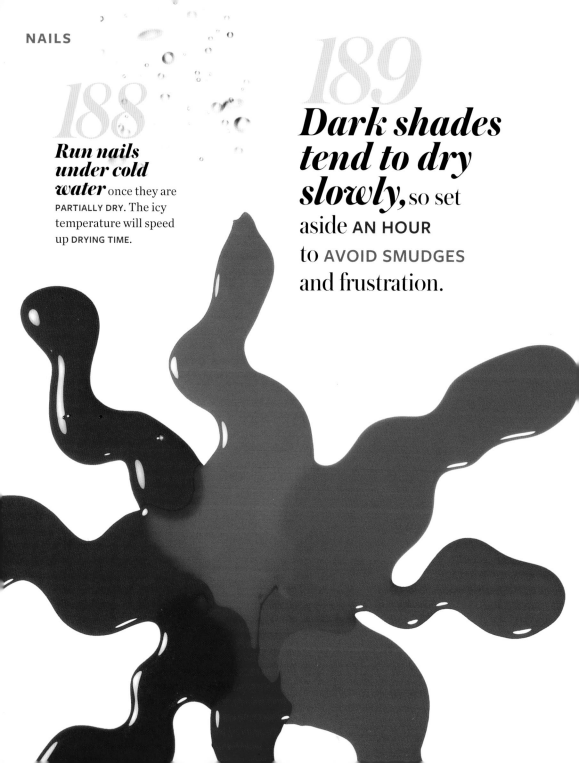

188

Run nails under cold water once they are PARTIALLY DRY. The icy temperature will speed up DRYING TIME.

189

Dark shades tend to dry slowly, so set aside AN HOUR to AVOID SMUDGES and frustration.

190

"I LOVE THE LOOK OF BUFFED NAILS. THEY LOOK NEAT AND CHIC WITHOUT ACTUALLY HAVING TO PAINT YOUR NAILS—AND IT TAKES NO TIME!"
—JOY BRYANT

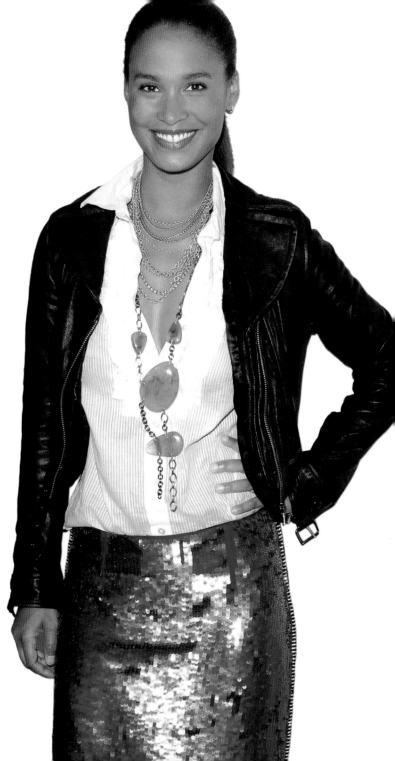

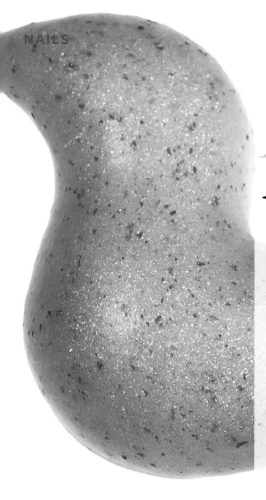

191

{ *3 ways to get rid of nail stains* }

1. Soak fingers in denture cleanser for about three minutes, suggests manicurist April Foreman, who has worked with Halle Berry and Jennifer Lopez. The liquid's oxidizing agents help bleach nails.

2. Take a break from polish for a month and use a two-sided buffer once a week to remove stains and restore shine.

3. For really stubborn stains, N.Y.C. nail guru Jin Soon Choi, owner of Jin Soon Natural Hand and Foot spas, recommends dabbing whitening toothpaste onto nail beds. "The whitening agents work on nails the same way they do on teeth."

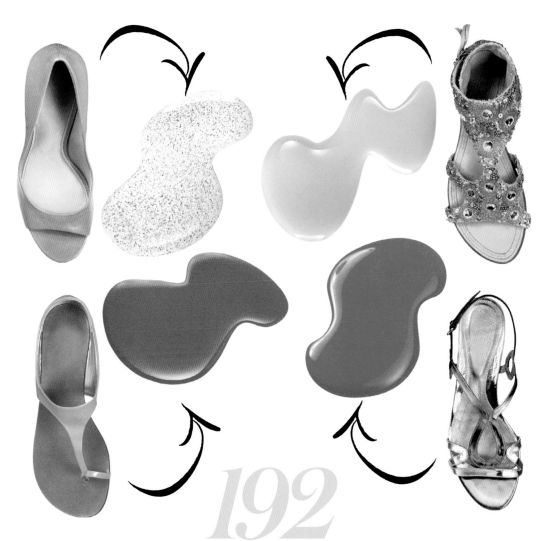

192

Think about your shoes when picking a pedicure color. Ji Baek, owner of Rescue Beauty Lounge in N.Y.C., says, "The MORE EMBELLISHED the sandal, the MORE NEUTRAL TOES should be. No metallic with metallic. Be daring with polish when wearing conservative shoes. And coral goes with anything!"

193

In warm weather, "the most common problem is cracked, dry heels from wearing sandals," says Jin Soon Choi. She recommends that you get into the habit of slathering on a thick foot cream after showering, when skin is most receptive. "To heal cracks, *use a rich foot balm*," she suggests. And, once a week, indulge in a relaxing lavender mineral soak to reduce swelling, followed by *an invigorating peppermint-and-pumice scrub*. During the day, keep a stash of cleansing towelettes in your purse or desk drawer to wipe grime off sandal-weary feet.

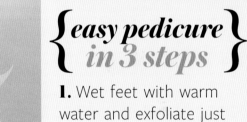

Use alcohol- and acetone-free nail-polish removers to take off lighter polish shades. While acetones are the most effective, they are also THE MOST DRYING, so save them for REMOVING DARK colors.

194

195

{ *easy pedicure* } { *in 3 steps* }

1. Wet feet with warm water and exfoliate just corns and calluses with a dab of body scrub.

2. File nails into a square shape.

3. Brush on a light-colored polish and a top coat. With light colors it doesn't matter if you don't have a super-steady hand.

Q&A

BURNING QUESTIONS, FINALLY ANSWERED

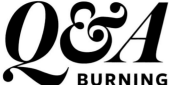

I WANT TO GET RID OF THE AGE SPOTS ON MY HANDS. WHAT ARE MY OPTIONS?

Sun damage causes melanin, the pigment in skin, to concentrate in brown spots. The first step: Stop further damage by wearing a hand cream containing sunblock every single day. A cream with a bleaching agent such as hydroquinone or kojic acid can lighten existing spots. As a last resort, you can try laser treatments. During the treatment, pulses of light from the laser cause the pigment to heat up, darken, and shatter.

IS IT TRUE THAT EATING GELATIN OR TAKING CALCIUM WILL STRENGTHEN MY NAILS?

Gelatin is a protein, and a severely protein-deprived diet weakens nails. But gelatin will benefit nails only if you have a deficiency. Calcium strengthens bones, but it isn't an integral part of nail structure. Your best bet: Take 2.5 milligrams daily of biotin, a B-complex vitamin that has been shown to strengthen nails.

HOW CAN I STOP BITING

MY NAILS? Try to keep your nails polished at all times—the brighter the color, the better. Applying cuticle oil daily can also inhibit biting because it's hard to get a grip on a slippery surface. To up the ante, keep a weekly standing appointment with a manicurist and tell her you're trying to kick the habit. You'll be less likely to destroy a perfect manicure (that you paid for), and she can offer you moral support.

HOW DO I KNOW IF I HAVE A NAIL INFECTION? WHAT CAN I DO TO PREVENT ONE AND MAKE SURE THAT MY MANICURE IS HYGIENIC?

If you have redness, swelling and pain around your nails, you probably

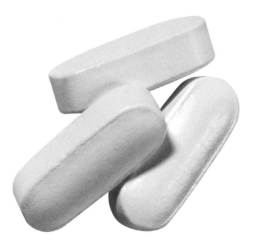

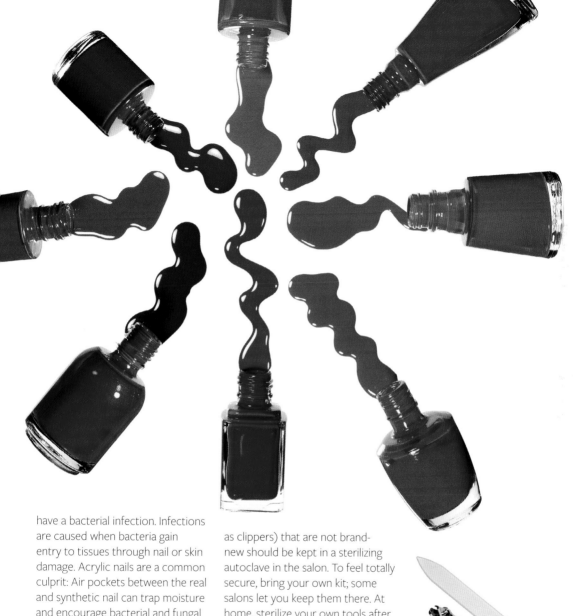

have a bacterial infection. Infections are caused when bacteria gain entry to tissues through nail or skin damage. Acrylic nails are a common culprit: Air pockets between the real and synthetic nail can trap moisture and encourage bacterial and fungal growth. Even regular manicures, if they're not done hygienically, can cause infections. Make sure your manicurist always uses a new emery board. Any salon tools (such as clippers) that are not brand-new should be kept in a sterilizing autoclave in the salon. To feel totally secure, bring your own kit; some salons let you keep them there. At home, sterilize your own tools after every use by placing them in boiling water for 10 minutes, then wiping them with alcohol. To avoid fungal infections, be sure salon soaking basins are disinfected between uses.

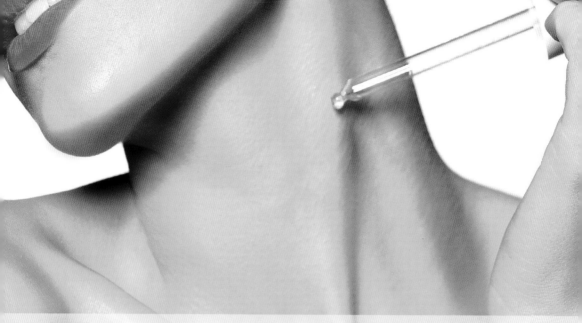

The Best of the Rest

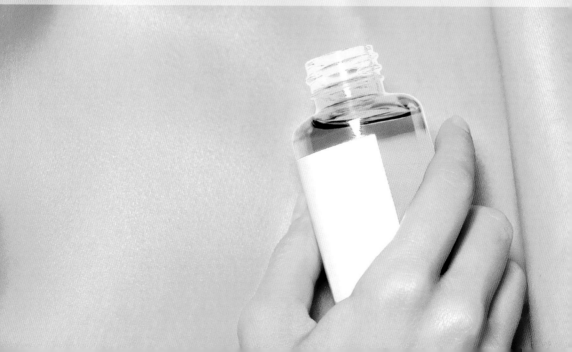

Know your scents

196

When picking a perfume, don't
judge a scent at first sniff. It takes about 10 MINUTES for the fragrance's "heart," the part that lasts the longest, to develop fully, says perfumer Frédéric Malle.

197

Scent lasts longer on well-hydrated skin,
so MOISTURIZE first with an UNSCENTED LOTION (and let it absorb) before putting on fragrance.

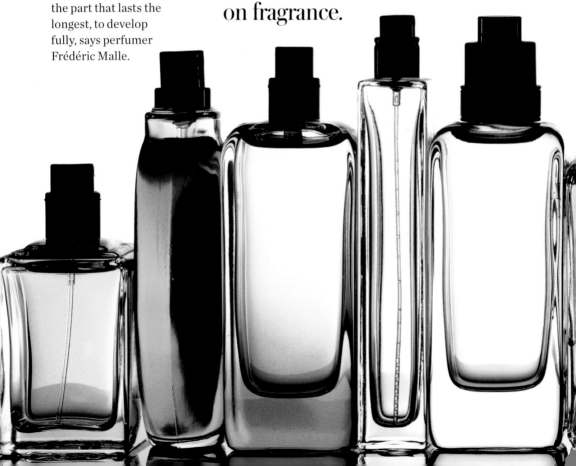

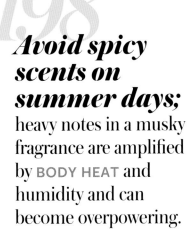

198

Avoid spicy scents on summer days; heavy notes in a musky fragrance are amplified by BODY HEAT and humidity and can become overpowering.

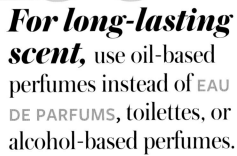

199

For long-lasting scent, use oil-based perfumes instead of EAU DE PARFUMS, toilettes, or alcohol-based perfumes.

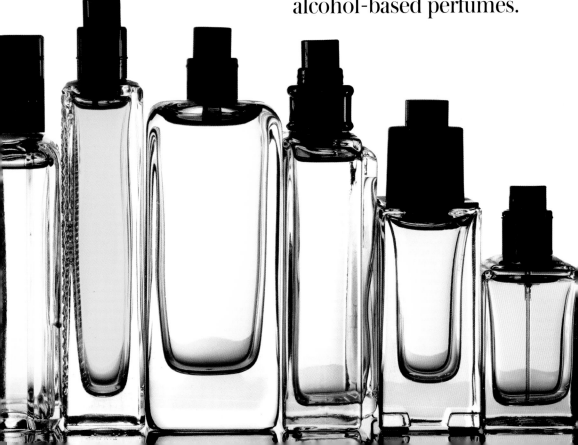

Know your scents

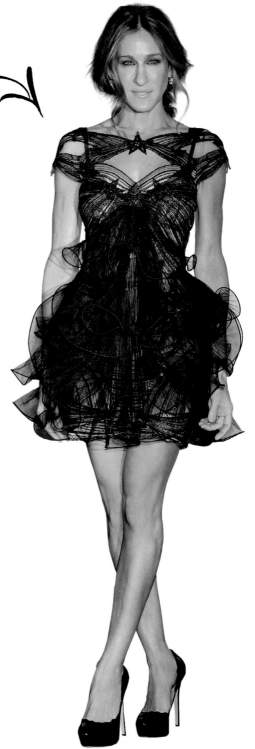

200

"I LOVE WALKING INTO A CLOSET AND SMELLING LINGERING PERFUME, SO I ALWAYS SPRAY MY CLOTHES. AND AT THE END OF THE BOTTLE, WHEN THE ATOMIZER NO LONGER REACHES THE TINY LITTLE DRIBBLE THAT IS LEFT, I UNSCREW THE TOP AND POUR THE REMAINDER ONTO A T-SHIRT OR DRESS."
—SARAH JESSICA PARKER

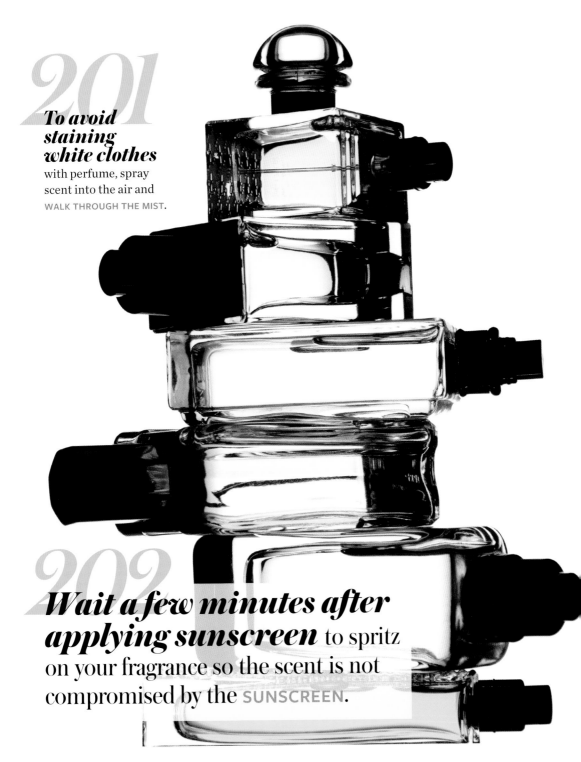

201

To avoid staining white clothes with perfume, spray scent into the air and WALK THROUGH THE MIST.

202

Wait a few minutes after applying sunscreen to spritz on your fragrance so the scent is not compromised by the SUNSCREEN.

Master the no-makeup look

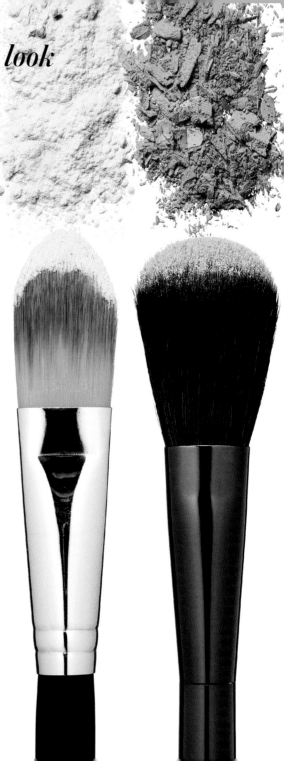

203

{ *minimal* *makeup magic* }

Get a "natural beauty" glow in six steps, thanks to N.Y.C. makeup artist Rie Omoto, who has worked with Rachel Bilson and Portia de Rossi.

1. Prep skin with liquid foundation and concealer, applying foundation first, blending with a brush, and rubbing in concealer with your fingers where needed.

2. Use subtle blush shades to emphasize your bone structure: Brush a darker blush in the hollow of your cheeks up to your temples, then dust cheeks with a lighter shade.

3. Use an eye shadow brush to apply a neutral shadow in the creases of your eyes and along your lower lash lines.

4. Stroke a shimmery version of the neutral shadow on the center of your upper lids (below the crease) and in the corners of your eyes to catch the light.

5. Fill in lips with a pencil that matches your lip color, then apply sheer peachy pink gloss with a lip brush.

Achieve an allover glow

204

For a sexy décolletage, first exfoliate your chest area with a moisturizing body scrub, says N.Y.C. dermatologist Anne Chapas. Then apply SHIMMERY LOTION from the clavicle down, followed by A DAB OF CREAM HIGHLIGHTER over the tops of the breasts. Finish with a dusting of BRONZING POWDER in the center of your chest; layer the color softly, then blend well.

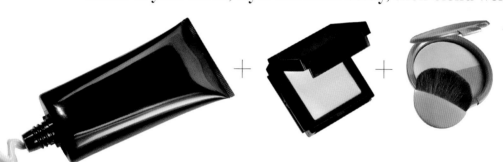

205

Warm up arms by using a bronzing body lotion or gel, or for a lighter shade, mix body bronzer or shimmer lotion with your REGULAR MOISTURIZER. Just be sure not to use facial bronzer on your body. Makeup artist Nick Barose, who has worked with Kerry Washington and Maria Bello, warns, "Makeup for the face may RUB OFF ON CLOTHES."

Achieve an allover glow

206 **Give legs a light, natural glow** by using self-tanner. Mix just a dab with your REGULAR LOTION and apply.

207

Make legs look extra svelte by misting skin with tinted spray for a golden glow, then brushing SHIMMERY POWDER straight down the front and back of legs. "Don't brush it all the way around," advises makeup pro Linda Hay, who preps the VICTORIA'S SECRET ANGELS. "This gives the illusion of a more streamlined shape."

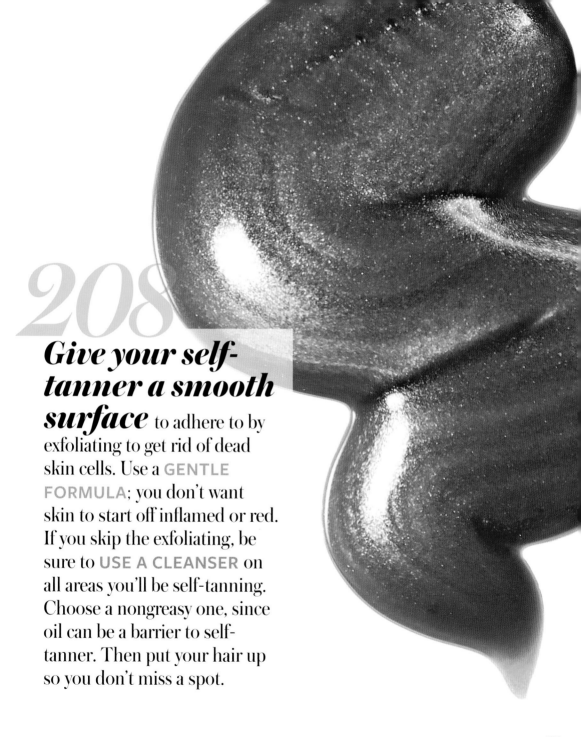

208

Give your self-tanner a smooth surface to adhere to by exfoliating to get rid of dead skin cells. Use a GENTLE FORMULA; you don't want skin to start off inflamed or red. If you skip the exfoliating, be sure to USE A CLEANSER on all areas you'll be self-tanning. Choose a nongreasy one, since oil can be a barrier to self-tanner. Then put your hair up so you don't miss a spot.

Self-tan perfectly

209

Apply undereye cream so that your tan will appear lighter below your eyes; you look younger when this area is brighter, says Jennifer Lopez's makeup artist Scott Barnes. Also rub an OINTMENT (LIKE VASELINE) on your cuticles and nails so you won't stain your fingertips OR RUIN YOUR POLISH.

210

Make sure your skin is hydrated. Slather on a light moisturizer all over. You can apply self-tanner while SKIN IS STILL MOIST from lotion—which will dilute the intensity of the tanner and decrease your chance of streaking—or wait until your SKIN IS DRY to the touch to avoid any interference with the tanner.

211

Apply tanner from the bottom up, beginning

with one light coat. Going from the bottom up works best since doing it in the OPPOSITE DIRECTION means you might get lines across your belly when you bend over to reach your legs. Use a paddle applicator for hard-to-reach spots like your back and shoulders.

212

Blast skin with a blow-dryer after you finish. The heat

helps the formula dry more quickly so it's less likely to stain your clothes. AVOID EXERCISE for eight hours to let the product sink in; sweat will create streaks, says makeup artist Torsten Witte.

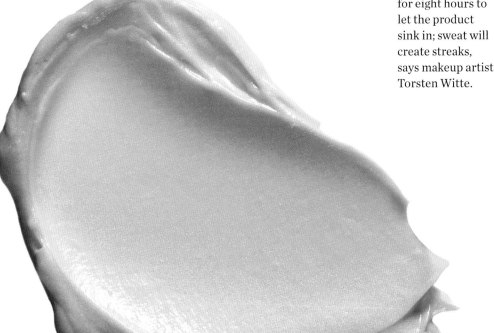

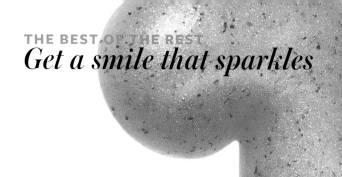

213

Reduce the presence of stain-causing acids in your mouth with a whitening toothpaste that contains peroxide and baking soda, which neutralizes acid, says N.Y.C. aesthetic dentist Jonathan Levine, who has worked on Sarah Jessica Parker and Kate Winslet. For STUBBORN STAINS, try a peroxide rinse and an at-home whitening or bleaching kit. Use them for only about 10 days, though; if you bleach teeth for months instead of weeks, you can damage them, making your smile look "BLUE TRANSPARENT," says Levine.

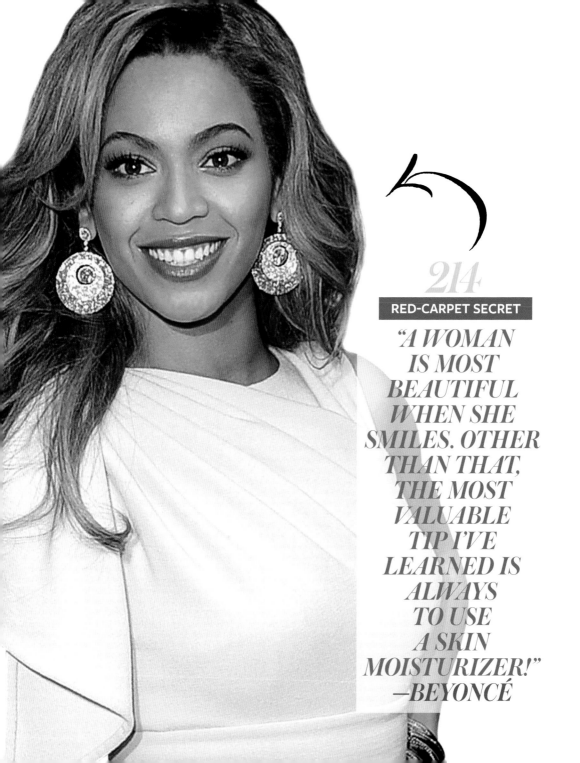

RED-CARPET SECRET

"A WOMAN IS MOST BEAUTIFUL WHEN SHE SMILES. OTHER THAN THAT, THE MOST VALUABLE TIP I'VE LEARNED IS ALWAYS TO USE A SKIN MOISTURIZER!"
—BEYONCÉ

Don't forget to toss old makeup

215

The more you touch a product, the faster it will acquire bacteria. Foundation in a pump bottle or a tube can be USED UNTIL IT'S FINISHED, but a pot of concealer should be REPLACED AFTER SIX MONTHS.

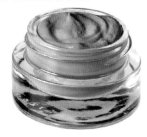

216

Mascara and eyeliner should be tossed after three months since they are EASILY CONTAMINATED by bacteria from your eyes.

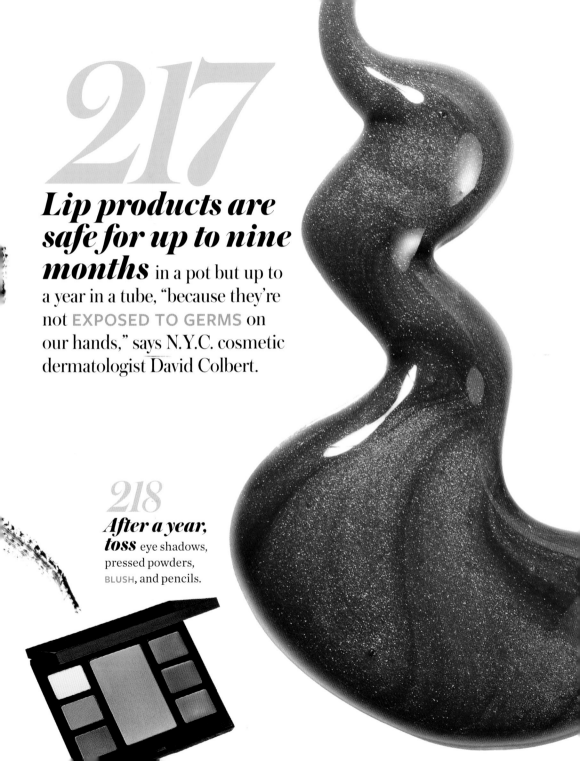

217

Lip products are safe for up to nine months in a pot but up to a year in a tube, "because they're not EXPOSED TO GERMS on our hands," says N.Y.C. cosmetic dermatologist David Colbert.

218

After a year, toss eye shadows, pressed powders, BLUSH, and pencils.

Q&A
BURNING QUESTIONS, FINALLY ANSWERED

I WANT MY SMILE TO LOOK RADIANT AT MY WEDDING. HOW CAN I GET MY TEETH THEIR BRIGHTEST?

For a truly white wedding, go for a power bleaching two weeks prior. "We use a strong concentration of hydrogen peroxide and put teeth under a white light," explains N.Y.C. dentist Gregg Lituchy. "It penetrates through the enamel to the dentin— the inner tooth structure—where it breaks apart stains." Be careful for the next two weeks: "The teeth are still porous, so stains are more likely to seep in." That means avoid coffee, tea, and red wine.

MY SKIN GETS DRY AND BUMPY AFTER I SHAVE MY LEGS. HOW CAN I PREVENT THIS?

If you're using a foaming shave cream or bar soap to help get stubble-free, that would explain the irritation. "They can be very drying," says N.Y.C. dermatologist Susan Binder. She recommends a non-foaming formula or a mild cleanser, like Cetaphil, for extra moisture. The proper technique is also important. For the gentlest removal, Binder suggests using a razor with no more than two blades and says to "always shave in the direction of hair growth."

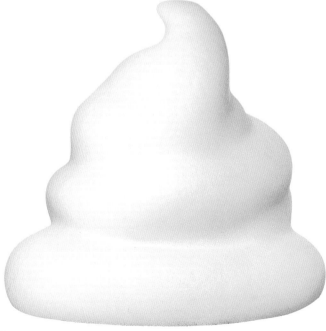

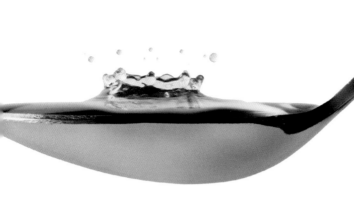

I'M CONFUSED BY THE SEALS ON THE NATURAL AND ORGANIC PRODUCTS I BUY. WHAT SHOULD I LOOK FOR?

The USDA Organic seal guarantees that at least 95 percent of the ingredients are organic or grown without synthetic chemicals. The Natural Product Association (NPA) seal certifies that 95 percent of the ingredients are natural or naturally derived, and there are no additives that pose a health risk. Ecocert is another seal to look for. Products stamped with this label are at least 95 percent organic. Ecocert is regulated by the USDA and oversees organic products in more than 80 countries.

I WASH MY HANDS A LOT IN THE WINTER TO KEEP FROM GETTING SICK, BUT NOW THEY'RE ALWAYS DRY AND SENSITIVE. HELP!

First things first: Wash your hands with warm water instead of hot, which can overstrip the skin's natural oils and leave it dehydrated, says N.Y.C. dermatologist Neal Schultz. After drying hands, apply cream containing moisturizing ingredients such as shea butter, glycerin, and aloe. If skin gets red and irritated, try this DIY remedy: Soak a cotton handkerchief in a solution of a half cup skim milk and a half cup water. Wring it out and place it on your skin for five to 10 minutes. "The protein in the milk heals the chafing and dryness," says Schultz.

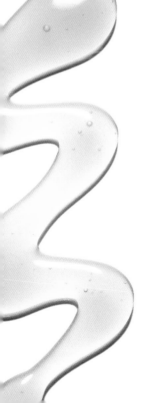

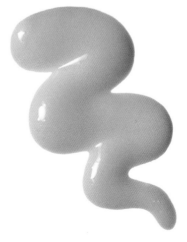

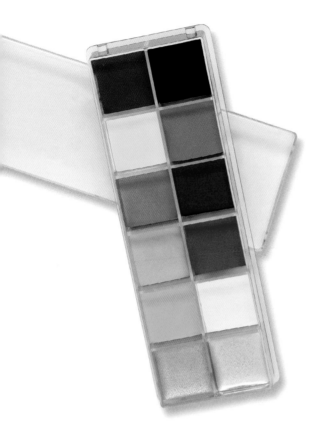

Beauty Buzzwords

Don't know your AHAs from your UVBs? Check out our glossary of tricky makeup and skin-care terms to make beauty jargon as simple as ABC (that's Antioxidants, Bioflavonoids and Collagen).

ABLATIVE/NON-ABLATIVE LASERS These heat lasers are used to treat scarring (often from acne or sun damage) and to resurface the skin to diminish wrinkles and improve pigmentation. Ablative lasers are more aggressive, removing the outer layer of skin to treat scarring; non-ablative lasers keep the epidermis intact and are used to treat more superficial scarring and facial wrinkles, especially in delicate areas such as around the eyes.

ALPHA HYDROXY ACIDS (AHAs) Natural chemical compounds that are often derived from fruit, AHAs help exfoliate dead skin and combat aging. Common AHAs found in skin-care products include glycolic acid, lactic acid, and citric acid.

ANTIOXIDANTS These chemical compounds slow the oxidation of cells by preventing the formation of free radicals, which cause cells to age and degrade (think of what happens when an apple slice is exposed to air). Used as ingredients in skin-care products, antioxidants may be natural, such as vitamins C and E and beta carotene, or synthetic, such as BHT (butylated hydroxytoluene).

BENZOYL PEROXIDE Found in cleansers, gels, creams and lotions, this is one of the most frequently used ingredients to treat acne. The bacteria that cause acne breakouts can't survive in the presence of oxygen; benzoyl peroxide releases oxygen into the pores, killing bacteria and causing the skin to dry and peel, opening blocked pores.

BETA HYDROXY ACIDS BHAs are similar to AHAs in that they exfoliate skin and encourage cell renewal. They are fat-soluble, so they can penetrate oil-filled pores, and are often prescribed for acne. Salicylic acid is a BHA.

BIOFLAVONOIDS Derived from fruits and vegetables, bioflavonoids are thought to have antioxidant properties and work with vitamin C to promote healthy collagen and capillaries.

CERAMIDES These natural fats (lipids) exist in the skin to help it retain moisture. Many creams use synthetic ceramides to plump skin and fight aging.

CO-ENZYME Q10 A naturally occurring antioxidant that also helps the skin's cellular respiratory system to function, co-enzyme Q10 starts to diminish after age 30, making it harder to produce collagen and elastin.

COLLAGEN One of the main proteins in skin and connective tissue, collagen binds with water, keeping skin looking plump and healthy. The production of collagen fibers decreases with age, causing wrinkles to appear.

CUTICLE This term is used both for nails (to describe the flap of skin at the base of the fingernail) and hair (for the protective outer layer of the hair shaft). When cuticles are healthy, nails and hair are strong and shiny. But if the cuticles in hair are damaged by chemicals, heat, or overprocessing, dullness and breakage can result.

DEPILATORY Depilation is the removal of unwanted hair from the face or body by any means, including shaving or waxing. But a depilatory refers specifically to a chemical sulfide that dissolves hair in the follicle.

DHA Dihydroxyacetone is the active ingredient in sunless tanners. A glycerol derivative, it reacts with amino acids and oxidizes just the surface of skin, giving it a tanned appearance without the damage associated with UV exposure.

DIMETHICONE This organic silicone is a common skin-care ingredient that creates a film on the skin's surface to retain moisture and plump fine lines.

ELASTIN Collagen's partner-in-beauty, elastin is another fibrous connective tissue found in skin. But while collagen gives skin firmness, elastin makes it supple.

EMULSIFIER A thickener or binding agent, this unifier joins two or more ingredients in a way that alters their physical makeup, for example, by thickening a lotion into a cream. In food, egg yolk is a common emulsifier; in a beauty product, it's likely to be cetearyl alcohol or an emulsifying wax.

FREE RADICALS These scavenging molecules, found in the environment and also produced by our bodies, cause cell breakdown and inflammation that can lead to disease and wrinkled skin. Antioxidants help fight their effects.

GLYCOLIC ACID A plant-derived alpha hydroxy acid (also known as hydroxyacetic acid), this substance exfoliates skin and is used to fight acne, wrinkles, and discoloration and promote cell renewal.

GRAPE-SEED EXTRACT A powerful antioxidant and bioflavonoid, this ingredient helps fight free radicals and improve circulation and skin elasticity.

HUMECTANT Any ingredient—such as glycerin—that pulls moisture from the surrounding air into the skin or hair, increasing its moisture retention, is known as a humectant.

HYALURONIC ACID A naturally occurring substance that retains moisture in the skin, hyaluronic acid is used as both a cosmetic filler and an ingredient in skin-care products. In the latter, it fights skin dehydration by plumping cells and temporarily reducing the appearance of fine lines.

HYPERPIGMENTATION This is a condition in which patches of skin

become darkened when UV rays provoke melanocytes (see entry) to create extra melanin. Hormones can make skin more prone to hyperpigmentation. It is often treated with topical lightening agents such as vitamin C or hydroquinone, or with lasers.

HYPOALLERGENIC This term is used to indicate ingredients or products that are unlikely to cause allergic reactions. The use of this term is not overseen by the FDA, however, so it's best to scan a product's ingredients list (which every product is required to display) to see if you are allergic to anything on it.

KERATIN An extremely strong protein, this amino acid is a key component in healthy hair, skin, and nails, and is used in many beauty products.

LACTIC ACID A widely used alpha hydroxy acid that is derived from milk, lactic acid is used as an exfoliant to help soften rough skin; it also helps skin retain moisture.

LED TREATMENTS LED stands for light-emitting diode. Specific wavelengths of light are aimed at the face to treat acne (blue LEDs kill skin bacteria) or sun damage (red LEDs boost skin cells' energy, stimulating regeneration). Treatments may be done in a doctor's office, or by the patient at home, using a handheld device.

LIPOSOMES A liposome is a microscopic delivery system created in a lab; its outer walls are made of lipids similar to those found in skin, but the interior can hold any ingredient for delivery. It is commonly used to deliver active ingredients to the skin.

MELANOCYTE A cell that produces pigment (also called melanin) and is responsible for the color in your hair, skin, and eyes. The darker your skin, the more melanin you have.

MICRO-ENCAPSULATION Through this process, tiny particles are coated and turned into spherical microcapsules. Active ingredients that biodegrade quickly become more stable if they are micro-encapsulated because the ingredient inside is protected.

PABA Para-aminobenzoic acid is a UV-absorbing chemical sunscreen that causes reactions in some users, so it is no longer found in most sunblocks. If you have sensitive skin, check the label and ingredients list to be sure a product is PABA-free.

PEPTIDES These groups of amino acids combine to form proteins, such as collagen, which keep skin firm. Naturally occurring in skin, they are also found in many skin-care products.

pH This is used to measure the acidity and basicity of a solution or a cosmetic. "pH-balanced" means neutral (and is the ideal that many cosmetic products aim for). A neutral substance (like water or milk) will have a pH of 7. Acidic substances have a pH value below 7, and base or alkali substances have a pH higher than 7.

PHOTOAGING The visible result of sun damage, photoaging refers to the premature breakdown of skin cells caused by UVA and UVB damage. In terms of your appearance, that means wrinkles, slackness, and discoloration.

PHOTOSENSITIVITY Essentially, this is sun sensitivity. It's the reason rashes, swelling, or pigment problems occur after sun exposure. It can be triggered by certain chemicals, drugs, foods, or the application of vitamin A. Also, certain ingredients, like retinol and chemical sunscreens like Avobenzone, are photosensitive; that is, they break down (are destabilized) when exposed to sun.

PHTHALATES Organic chemicals used as plasticizers, phthalates are found in most nail polish (they make it harder and more durable) and perfume (they make it last longer). Government agencies have ruled that phthalates are safe in the small doses in which they occur in beauty products, but because these chemicals have been shown to affect sex hormones, some people prefer to use products that are phthalate-free.

POLYPHENOLS A group of anti-oxidants found in substances such as green tea and grape seeds, they're also used in topical skin creams for their free-radical-fighting benefit.

RESTYLANE A hyaluronic-acid-based injectable dermatological filler, Restylane is used to re-sculpt the face, for example, filling wrinkles and plumping lips.

RETINOIDS These powerful chemical compounds derived from vitamin A are often used to treat acne, increase collagen formation, and even out skin pigment. They may appear on product labels as tretinoin, retinoic acid, or retinol.

SERUM Technically, a serum is the clear or watery part of any bodily fluid. In terms of beauty products, serum often refers to a fluid that is lighter than a lotion and rich in active ingredients. To get the full benefit, you apply it before you put on other, thicker products.

SPF Sun Protection Factor is a measure of how long your skin can stay in the sun without burning. SPF measures the effect of only UVB rays (see entry), which cause burning. The FDA is developing a more comprehensive sunblock rating system; in the meantime, look for a product that offers broad-spectrum protection (from UVA and UVB rays).

SULFATE Any chemical compound containing sulfur that acts as a detergent can be called a sulfate. Sodium lauryl sulfate and ammonium lauryl sulfate, for example, can be found in household cleansers, toothpastes, shampoos, and conditioners. Studies have indicated that sulfates may irritate skin and build up in body tissue, so some consumers prefer sulfate-free alternatives.

SURFACTANT Also known as a surface-acting agent, a surfactant lowers the tension of a liquid, making it combine more easily with other substances. In beauty products, surfactants are often foaming agents or lubricants, as in shaving cream.

THERMAGE A noninvasive treatment using radio frequency, thermage consists of a dermatologist's exposing a patient's skin to radio-wave pulses of heat to stimulate and thicken collagen and make skin appear tighter and smoother.

UVA/UVB The UV stands for ultraviolet. Ultraviolet light is made up of the invisible rays of sunlight that cause burns, photoaging, and skin cancer. Type A UV rays, with their long wavelengths, penetrate skin deeply and cause photoaging. Type B UV rays, whose wavelengths are shorter, visibly and quickly damage the outer layers of skin, causing dryness, redness, tanning, and burns. Think of them as UVAging and UVBurning.

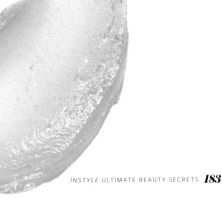

Our Experts

Kimara Ahnert, owner of Kimara Ahnert Studio, N.Y.C.

Lisa Airan, aesthetic dermatologist, Lisa Airan, M.D., N.Y.C.; clinical professor of dermatology, Mount Sinai Hospital, N.Y.C.

Tina Alster, founding director, Washington Institute of Dermatologic Laser Surgery, Washington, D.C.

Jan Arnold, co-founder, Creative Nail Design

Billy B., makeup artist

Ji Baek, owner, Rescue Beauty Lounge, N.Y.C.

Jake Bailey, makeup artist

John Bailey, chief scientist, Personal Care Products Council

David Bank, founding director, Center for Dermatology, Cosmetic and Laser Surgery , Mount Kisco, N.Y.

Scott Barnes, makeup artist

Nick Barose, makeup artist

Cristina Bartolucci, makeup artist and co-founder, DuWop Cosmetics

Gita Bass, makeup artist

Leslie Baumann, dermatologist and CEO, Baumann Cosmetic and Research Institute, Miami Beach

Regine Bedot, makeup artist

Kenneth Beer, dermatologist and founder, Scientific by Kenneth Beer, M.D.

Susan Binder, dermatologist, N.Y.C.

Paco Blancas, makeup artist

Monika Blunder, makeup artist

Fredric Brandt, dermatologist, N.Y.C. and Coral Gables, Fla., and founder, Dr. Brandt Skincare

Gina Brooke, artistic director, Hourglass Cosmetics and Intraceuticals

Jaimi Brooks, founder, Fiore Beauty

Bobbi Brown, founder, Bobbi Brown Cosmetics

Tasha Reiko Brown, makeup artist

Kara Yoshimoto Bua, makeup artist, Chanel

Kristofer Buckle, makeup artist

Patty Bunch, owner, The Bungalow Skin Therapy Spa

Linda Cantello, makeup artist, Giorgio Armani Beauty

Carmindy, makeup artist, *What Not to Wear*, and co-creator, Sally Hansen Natural Beauty Inspired by Carmindy

Anne Chapas, dermatologist, Laser and Skin Surgery Center of New York, N.Y.C.

Gabriel Chiu, plastic surgeon, Beverly Hills Plastic Surgery, Inc., Beverly Hills

Jin Soon Choi, founder, Jin Soon Natural Hand and Foot Spa, N.Y.C.

Lauren Kaye Cohen, makeup artist

David Colbert, founder and head physician, New York Dermatology Group, N.Y.C.

Colleen Creighton, makeup artist

Nonie Creme, founding creative director, Butter London

AJ Crimson, co-founder, Kissable Couture Lipgloss and Beauty Statements by AJ Crimson

Joanna Czech, aesthetician and owner, Sava Spa, N.Y.C.

Sonya Dakar, aesthetician and founder, Sonya Dakar Skin Clinic, Beverly Hills

Maggie Ford Danielson, global trend makeup artist, Benefit

Steeve Daviault, makeup artist, Lancôme

Doris Day, founder and director, Day Dermatology and Aesthetics, N.Y.C.

Mario Dedivanovic, makeup artist

Aaron De Mey, artistic director, Lancôme

Jillian Dempsey, makeup artist, Avon

Sue Devitt, founder, Sue Devitt Beauty

Paula Dorf, founder, Paula Dorf Cosmetics

Mimi Dorsey, founder, Unique Image Design Consulting

Dotti, makeup artist, Nars Cosmetics

Jeffrey Dover, dermatologist and associate clinical professor of dermatology, Yale University

Pati Dubroff, makeup artist

Elle, manicurist, Barielle

April Foreman, manicurist

Robin Fredriksz, makeup artist

Brett Freedman, makeup artist

Francesca Fusco, assistant clinical professor of dermatology, Mount Sinai School of Medicine, N.Y.C.

Carl Geffken, vice president, Independent Cosmetic Manufacturers and Distributors

Lee Graff, president and co-creator, Cover FX

Charlie Green, makeup artist

Dennis Gross, dermatologist and founder, Dr. Dennis Gross Skin Care

Melanie Grossman, dermatologist, N.Y.C.

Skyy Hadley, owner, As U Wish Nail Spa, Hoboken, N.J.

Kimberly Harms, dentist, Rivers Edge Dental Clinic, Farmington, Minn.

Linda Hay, makeup artist

Romero Jennings, senior artist, MAC Cosmetics

Troy Jensen, makeup artist, Jouer Cosmetics

Ashlie Johnson, manicurist

Nerida Joy, aesthetician and founder, Nerida Joy Skincare

Bruce Katz, dermatologist and director, Juva Skin and Laser Center, N.Y.C.

Arielle Kauvar, dermatologist and founder and director, New York Laser and Skin Care, N.Y.C.

Diane Kendal, makeup artist

Jemma Kidd, founder, Jemma Kidd Makeup School, Jemma Kidd Pro Brands, JK Jemma Kidd

Anthea King, makeup artist, Mark Cosmetics

Poppy King, founder, Lipstick Queen

Peter Kopelson, dermatologist and founder, Laser Aesthetics and Advanced Dermatology, Beverly Hills

Kate Lee, makeup artist, Chanel

Soul Lee, makeup artist, Shu Uemura

Lyn Leigh, consultant, the Fragrance Foundation

Angela Levin, makeup artist, Chanel

Jonathan Levine, dentist and creator, GoSmile products; program director, the Advanced Aesthetics Program, New York School of Dentistry, N.Y.C.

Suzanne Levine, podiatric surgeon, Institute Beauté, N.Y.C.

Deborah Lippmann, founder, Deborah Lippmann nail line

Gregg Lituchy, cosmetic dentist, Lowenberg and Lituchy, N.Y.C.

Jeanine Lobell, makeup artist, Kevyn Aucoin Beauty

Leslie Lopez, makeup artist

Debra Luftman, founder, Luftman MD dermatology, Beverly Hills; clinical instructor of dermatology and skin surgery, University of California, Los Angeles

Elissa Lunder, dermatologist, Dermatology Partners, Wellesley, Mass.

Frédéric Malle, founder, Editions de Parfums Frédéric Malle

Stéphane Marais, makeup artist

Ellen Marmur, chief of dermatologic and cosmetic surgery, Mount Sinai Medical Center, N.Y.C.

Lorenzo Martin, makeup artist

Tracie Martyn, aesthetician and co-founder, Tracie Martyn Skincare

Susan McCarthy, makeup artist, Giorgio Armani Beauty

Laura Mercier, founder, Laura Mercier Cosmetics

Chantel Miller, senior artist, MAC Cosmetics

Karan Mitchell, makeup artist

Kay Montano, makeup artist, Chanel

Bethany Newell, manicurist

Ted Ning, director, Lifestyles of Health and Sustainability Organization

Rie Omoto, makeup artist

Dick Page, artistic director, Shiseido

Shane Paish, makeup artist, Dior

Denise Pereau, makeup artist

Nicholas V. Perricone, founder, Perricone MD Skin Care

Peter Philips, global creative director, Chanel

Lisa Postma, manicurist, OPI

Tim Quinn, makeup artist, Giorgio Armani Beauty

Mai Quynh, makeup artist, Mark Cosmetics

Nolan Robert, founder, Nolan Robert Cosmetics

Damone Roberts, founder, Damone Roberts New York, N.Y.C.

Mally Roncal, founder, Mally Beauty

Vanessa Scali, makeup artist

Joanna Schlip, makeup artist, Physicians Formula and Red Carpet Kolour

Neal Schultz, cosmetic dermatologist, N.Y.C., and founder, DermTV

Ashunta Sheriff, makeup artist, Mary Kay

Sofia Shusterov, manicurist

Anastasia Soare, founder, Anastasia Beverly Hills, Beverly Hills

Howard Sobel, dermatologist and founder, Skin and Spa Cosmetic Surgery Center, N.Y.C.

Kate Somerville, founder, Kate Somerville Skin Health Experts, L.A.

Andrew Sotomayor, makeup artist

Molly R. Stern, makeup artist, Cover Girl

Fiona Stiles, makeup artist

Jo Strettell, makeup artist

Troy Surratt, makeup artist

Amy Tagliamonti, senior makeup artist, Gossip Girl

Francesca Tolot, makeup artist

Tina Turnbow, makeup artist

Maria Verel, makeup artist

Stacey Lyn Weinstein, owner, Once Upon a Bride hair and makeup agency, N.Y.C.

Scott Wells, plastic surgeon, N.Y.C.

Gucci Westman, global artistic director, Revlon

Patricia Wexler, dermatologic surgeon, Wexler Dermatology Group, and founder, Patricia Wexler M.D. Dermatology Skin Care

Ni'kita Wilson, cosmetics chemist, and vice president, Cosmetech Laboratories

Torsten Witte, makeup artist, Nars Cosmetics

Index

S

salicylic acid, 26, 53

scars, 36

scents

    avoiding clothes stains, 167

    choice of, 164, 165

    long-lasting, 165

    moisturizing and, 164

    sunscreen and, 167

seasons

    transitional, 41

    See also summer; winter

self-tanner, 170, 171-173

sensitive skin, 22, 37

serums, 20, 21, 22, 183

skin

    cleansing, 10-11, 21, 22, 37, 107

    determining type, 18

    red skin, 22, 26, 36, 45, 54, 81

    sensitive, 22, 37

    splotchy skin, 22, 54, 127

    sunburn, 35, 45

    See also combination skin; dry skin; normal skin; oily skin; sunscreen

skin-brightening, 24

skin-care regimens, time needed for, 20

skin-care treatment products, thinnest to thickest application, 18

smoky eye, 86, 91, 92, 96, 100

special occasion secrets

    fake eyelashes, 106

    masks, 19

    primer, 48

SPF, 10, 46, 47, 183

splotchy skin, 22, 54, 127

sponges, 43

sulfates, 183

sulfur, 53

summer

    blush for, 61

    dry skin, 23

    eye tricks, 99

    feet tricks, 158

    foundation shades for, 41, 45

    lip tricks, 127

    scents for, 165

sunburn, 35, 45

sunscreen

    antioxidant day cream with, 21

    antioxidant serum before, 20

    application of, 33

    in foundation, 46

    for hands, 160

    irritation from, 33, 34

    for lightening foundation for winter, 47

    liquid bronzer in, 73

    melasma and, 36

    in moisturizers, 29, 37, 46

    neck versus face, 33

    scents and, 167

    skin cleansers for removing, 10

    sweat-proof sunblock, 48

    types of, 33, 34

sun spots, 36, 54

surfactant, 183

T

tanning, 151, 170, 171-173

teeth, 125, 126, 132, 174, 178

thermage, 183

throat, testing colors on, 41

titanium dioxide, 33

U

UVA/UVB, 35, 183

V

vitamin B3, 23

vitamin B5, 23

vitamin B-complex, 160

vitamin C, 11, 140

vitamin E, 20, 42

W

waxes, for facial fuzz, 13

whitening toothpaste, 156, 174

winter

    bronzer for, 75

    foundation shades for, 41, 47

    lip tricks, 137

    make-it-yourself humidifier, 31

    moisturizing nails, 153

witch hazel, 37

wrinkles

    antioxidant serum, 20

    concealer mixed with eye cream, 51

    foundation application and, 43

    soy milk refresher, 24

    three steps for, 21

Y

yeast levels, 11

Z

zinc oxide, 33

Photography Credits

Front cover, clockwise from top left: Henry Leutwyler (2), Brian Henn/Time Inc. Digital Studio, Henry Leutwyler

Back cover, clockwise from top left: Svend Lindbaek (2), Henry Leutwyler, Brian Henn/Time Inc Digital Studio, Svend Lindbaek (2)

pp. 6-7, clockwise from top: Ryann Cooley, Dawn Giarrizzo/Time Inc. Digital Studio, Brian Henn/Time Inc. Digital Studio, Grant Cornett/Time Inc. Digital Studio

p. 9: Walter Chin/Trunk Archive

pp. 10-11: Time Inc. Digital Studio (3)

p. 12: Steve Granitz/WireImage

p. 13: Todd Huffman

pp. 14–15, from left to right: Brian Henn/Time Inc. Digital Studio, Jeff Harris

p. 16: Todd Huffman

p. 17: Jamie McCarthy/WireImage

p. 18: Brian Henn/Time Inc. Digital Studio (2)

p. 20: Brian Henn/Time Inc. Digital Studio (2)

p. 21: Brian Henn/Time Inc. Digital Studio

p. 22, from left to right: Grant Cornett/Time Inc. Digital Studio, iStock

p. 24, from left to right: Lew Robertson/FoodPix/Getty, Todd Huffman

p. 25: Jamie McCarthy/WireImage

p. 26: Jeffrey Westbrook/Time Inc. Digital Studio

p. 27: Grant Cornett/Time Inc. Digital Studio

p. 28: Dan Kitwood/Getty

p. 29: Brian Henn/Time Inc. Digital Studio

p. 30: Time Inc. Digital Studio

p. 32: Pseudo Image/Shooting Star

p. 33, from left to right: Devon Jarvis, Grant Cornett/Time Inc. Digital Studio

p. 34: Brian Henn/Time Inc. Digital Studio

p. 35: iStock

p. 36: Brian Henn/Time Inc. Digital Studio

p. 37: Brian Henn/Time Inc. Digital Studio

p. 39: Masterfile

p. 40: Jeffrey Westbrook/Time Inc. Digital Studio

p. 41, from left to right: Time Inc. Digital Studio, Brian Henn/Time Inc. Digital Studio

p. 42: Time Inc. Digital Studio

p. 43: Marcocchi Giulio/SIPA

p. 44, from top to bottom: Brian Henn/Time Inc. Digital Studio, Grant Cornett/Time Inc. Digital Studio

p. 46, from left to right: Grant Cornett/Time Inc. Digital Studio, Brian Henn/Time Inc. Digital Studio

p. 48, from left to right: Jeffrey Westbrook/Time Inc. Digital Studio, Brian Henn/Time Inc. Digital Studio

p. 49: Gregorio T. Binuya/Everett Digital

p. 50, from top to bottom: Brian Henn/Time Inc. Digital Studio, Jeff Harris

p. 51, from left to right: Time Inc. Digital Studio, Brian Henn/Time Inc. Digital Studio

p. 52: Brian Henn/Time Inc. Digital Studio (2)

p. 53: Brian Henn/Time Inc. Digital Studio (2)

p. 54, from left to right: Jeffrey Westbrook/Time Inc. Digital Studio, David Stesner

p. 55: Brian Henn/Time Inc. Digital Studio

p. 56: Time Inc. Digital Studio (2)

p. 57: Brian Henn/Time Inc. Digital Studio (2)

p. 59: Robin Derrick/Trunk Archive

p. 60, from top to bottom: Sephora, Devon Jarvis

p. 63: Svend Lindbaek

p. 64, from left to right: Alexander Milligan/Time Inc. Digital Studio, Frazer Harrison/Getty

p. 65: Devon Jarvis

p. 66: Brian Henn/Time Inc. Digital Studio (2)

p. 67: Brian Henn/Time Inc. Digital Studio

p. 68: Brian Henn/Time Inc. Digital Studio

p. 69: Grant Cornett/Time Inc. Digital Studio

p. 70, from left to right: Jeff Harris, Time Inc. Digital Studio

p. 71: Grant Cornett/Time Inc. Digital Studio

p. 72: Gregg DeGuire/WireImage

p. 73: Grant Cornett/Time Inc. Digital Studio

p. 74, from left to right: Grant Cornett/Time Inc. Digital Studio, Brian Henn/Time Inc. Digital Studio

p. 76: Alexander Milligan/Time Inc. Digital Studio

p. 77: Jean-Paul Aussen/WireImage

p. 78: Brian Henn/Time Inc. Digital Studio

p. 79, clockwise from top left: Todd Huffman (2), Mike Coppola/FilmMagic

p. 80: Time Inc. Digital Studio

p. 81: Henry Leutwyler

p. 83: Lorenzo Bringheli/Trunk Archive

p. 84: Jeffrey Westbrook (2)

p. 85, clockwise from left: Jeffrey Westbrook (2), Time Inc. Digital Studio

p. 86: Ron Wolfson/Zuma

p. 87, from top to bottom: Time Inc. Digital Studio, Brian Henn/Time Inc. Digital Studio

p. 88: Svend Lindbaek

p. 89: Todd Huffman (3)

p. 90: Time Inc. Digital Studio

p. 91: Brian Henn/Time Inc. Digital Studio

p. 92: Brian Henn/ Time Inc. Digital Studio

p. 93, from top to bottom: Jeff Harris, Devon Jarvis

p. 94: Jordan Strauss/Getty

p. 95, from left to right: Brian Henn/Time Inc. Digital Studio, Devon Jarvis, Brian Henn/Time Inc. Digital Studio

pp. 96–97, from left to right: Ryann Cooley, Jeff Harris

p. 98: Brian Henn/Time Inc. Digital Studio

p. 100: WENN

p. 101, from top to bottom: Todd Huffman, Jeffrey Westbrook/Time Inc. Digital Studio

p. 102: Todd Huffman

p. 103, from top to bottom: Time Inc. Digital Studio, iStock

p. 104. from left to right: Svend Lindbaek, Brian Henn/Time Inc. Digital Studio

p. 105: Brian Henn/Time Inc. Digital Studio

p. 107, from top to bottom: Henry Leutwyler, Time Inc. Digital Studio (4)

p. 108: Brian Hagiwara/FoodPix/Getty

p. 109: Grant Cornett/Time Inc. Digital Studio (2)

p. 110: Brian Henn/Time Inc. Digital Studio (2)

p. 111, from left to right: Todd Huffman, Brian Henn/Time Inc. Digital Studio

p. 112: David Livingston/Getty

p. 113: Brian Henn/Time Inc. Digital Studio (2)

p. 114, from left to right: Time Inc. Digital Studio, Don Penny/Time Inc. Digital Studio

p. 115: Brian Henn/Time Inc. Digital Studio

p. 117: Image Source/Lifesize/Getty

p. 118, from left to right: Time Inc. Digital Studio, Brian Henn/Time Inc. Digital Studio

p. 119: Pascal Le Segretain/Getty

p. 120: Grant Cornett/Time Inc. Digital Studio

p. 121: Grant Cornett/Time Inc. Digital Studio

p. 122: Brian Henn/Time Inc. Digital Studio

p. 123: Todd Huffman

p. 124: Brian Henn/Time Inc. Digital Studio (2)

p. 125: Byron Purvis/AdMedia

p. 126, from left to right: Svend Lindbaek, Grant Cornett/Time Inc. Digital Studio

p. 128: Dawn Giarrizzo/Time Inc. Digital Studio

p. 129: Brian Henn/Time Inc. Digital Studio

p. 130: Dimitrios Kambouris/WireImage

p. 131: Brian Henn/Time Inc. Digital Studio

p. 132: Brian Henn/Time Inc. Digital Studio

p. 133: Brian Henn/Time Inc. Digital Studio (2)

p. 134: Brian Henn/Time Inc. Digital Studio

p. 135: Svend Lindbaek

p. 136, from left to right: Time Inc. Digital Studio, Grant Cornett/Time Inc. Digital Studio

p. 138: Brian Henn/Time Inc. Digital Studio (2)

p. 139: Grant Cornett/Time Inc. Digital Studio

p. 140: Grant Cornett/Time Inc. Digital Studio

p. 141: Svend Lindbaek

p. 143: Ilan Rubin/Trunk Archive

p. 144, from top to bottom: Time Inc. Digital Studio, David Lewis Taylor

p. 145: Image Source/Alamy

p. 146: Kevin Cremens

p. 147, from left to right: Brian Henn/Time Inc. Digital Studio, David Lewis Taylor

p. 148, from left to right: Brian Henn/Time Inc. Digital Studio, Grant Cornett/Time Inc. Digital Studio

p. 149, from left to right: Todd Huffman, Grant Cornett/Time Inc. Digital Studio, Brian Henn/Time Inc. Digital Studio

p. 150: Nigel Cox

p. 151, from left to right: Time Inc. Digital Studio, Brian Henn/Time Inc. Digital Studio

p. 152, from left to right: Grant Cornett/Time Inc. Digital Studio, Brian Henn/Time Inc. Digital Studio

p. 154, from top to bottom: Hiroshi Watanabe/Getty, Jeffrey Westbrook/Time Inc. Digital Studio

p. 155: Craig Barritt/WireImage

p. 156: Brian Henn/Time Inc. Digital Studio

p. 157: Grant Cornett/Time Inc. Digital Studio

p. 159: Brian Henn/Time Inc. Digital Studio

p. 160: Grant Cornett/Time Inc. Digital Studio

p. 161, from left to right: Jeffrey Westbrook/Time Inc. Digital Studio, Time Inc. Digital Studio

p. 163: Graeme Montgomery/Trunk Archive

pp. 164–165: Buena Vista Images/Lifesize/Getty

p. 166: Tsuni/Gamma USA

p. 167: Buena Vista Images/Lifesize/Getty

p. 168: Svend Lindbaek

p. 169, from top to bottom: Grant Cornett/Time Inc. Digital Studio (3), Brian Henn/Time Inc. Digital Studio

p. 170: Brian Henn/Time Inc. Digital Studio

p. 171: Brian Henn/Time Inc. Digital Studio

p. 172: Brian Henn/Time Inc. Digital Studio

p. 173: Brian Henn/Time Inc. Digital Studio

p. 174: Brian Henn/Time Inc. Digital Studio

p. 175 Mejia Asadorian/Splash

p. 176, from left to right: Brian Henn/Time Inc. Digital Studio, iStock

p. 177, from left to right: Brian Henn/Time Inc. Digital Studio, Grant Cornett/Time Inc. Digital Studio

p. 178: Grant Cornett/Time Inc. Digital Studio

p. 179, clockwise from top: Momoko Takeda/Getty, Time Inc. Digital Studio, Brian Henn/Time Inc. Digital Studio

p. 180: David Lewis Taylor

p. 182: Jeffrey Westbrook/Time Inc. Digital Studio

p. 183: Brian Henn/Time Inc. Digital Studio